Suggestions
for Thought
by Florence
Nightingale

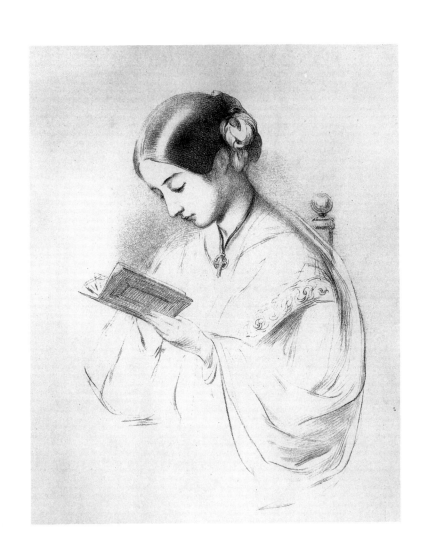

Suggestions for Thought
by Florence Nightingale

SELECTIONS AND
COMMENTARIES

Edited by
Michael D. Calabria and
Janet A. Macrae

PENN

University of Pennsylvania Press

Philadelphia

University of Pennsylvania Press
Studies in Health, Illness, and Caregiving
Joan E. Lynaugh, General Editor

A complete listing of the books in this series appears at the back of this volume

Copyright © 1994 by the University of Pennsylvania Press
Printed in the United States of America

Library of Congress Cataloging-in-Publication Data
Nightingale, Florence, 1820–1910.
   [Suggestions for thought to the searchers after truth among the artizans of England.
Selections]
   Selections for thought / by Florence Nightingale ; selections and commentaries edited by
Michael D. Calabria and Janet A. Macrae.
      p.   cm. — (University of Pennsylvania press studies of health, illness, and
caregiving)
   Includes bibliographical references and index.
   ISBN 0-8122-3174-0. — ISBN 0-8122-1501-X (pbk.)
   1. Religion.   2. Ethnics.   3. Nightingale, Florence, 1820–1910—Religion.   I. Calabria,
Michael D.   II. Macrae, Janet, 1947–   .   III. Title.   IV. Series.
BL50.N47   1994
291—dc20   93-37576
                                                                              CIP

10 9 8 7 6 5 4

Frontispiece: A lithograph of Florence Nightingale from a drawing by her cousin, Hilary
Bonham Carter. Reproduced courtesy of the Florence Nightingale Museum, London.

Contents

Preface

Florence Nightingale is best known as a woman of action: as the founder of modern nursing, a reformer in the field of public health, and a pioneer in the use of statistics. Her influence was so far-reaching that even the critical Lytton Strachey would write in 1918, ten years after her death, that "there is no great hospital today which does not bear upon it the impress of her mind."[1]

It is not generally known, however, that Nightingale was at the forefront of the religious and philosophical as well as the scientific thought of her time. In a three-volume work entitled *Suggestions for Thought*, Nightingale presented her radical spiritual views. Her motivation was to give those who had turned away from conventional religion an alternative to atheism.

Nightingale never published *Suggestions for Thought*, and very few biographers have discussed the work in any detail. This abridged and edited volume is thus designed to make the essence of Nightingale's spiritual philosophy accessible to the general public, as well as to scholars and students. As the original work was redundant in its 800 pages, we have selected the best-written treatments of all her major ideas and have reorganized them for ease of reading. In addition, we have provided an introduction and commentary to set the work into a biographical, historical, and philosophical context.

This work illuminates a little-known dimension of Nightingale's personality, bringing forth the ideas that served as guiding principles for her work. It is also a historical document as it deals with the religious issues that were fiercely debated in the second half of the nineteenth century. In many ways, however, much of it is surprisingly relevant today, when humanity is still trying to reconcile reason with faith. In *Suggestions for Thought*, one has the opportunity to experience one of the great practical minds of modern history as it grapples with the most profound questions of human existence. As these basic human issues are universal and timeless, Nightingale's words are as immediate and compelling now as they were over a century ago.

1. Strachey, *Eminent Victorians*, p. 162.

Because only a few copies were privately printed, *Suggestions for Thought* has been virtually inaccessible to all but the most persistent of researchers. The three volumes were issued on microfiche in 1981 by University Microfilms International as part of the Adelaide Nutting Historical Nursing Collection. We would like to thank David Ment, Head of Special Collections at Columbia University's Teacher's College, for granting us access to the copy in that collection.

In preparing this edition we have drawn from a number of manuscript collections. The largest collection of Nightingale's papers, letters, notes, and other documents are housed in the British Library. We would like to thank the Department of Manuscripts, British Library, for allowing us to consult these materials. Copyright of the Nightingale collection in the British Library is maintained by the Trustees of the Henry Bonham-Carter Will Trust. We would like to acknowledge the Trust for granting permission to quote from this material, and their solicitors Radcliffes & Co. for their assistance.

Another large collection of Nightingale's letters is located at Claydon House, Buckinghamshire, which was the home of Florence's sister Parthenope and her husband Sir Harry Verney. Photocopies of these letters are housed at the Wellcome Institute for the History of Medicine Library in London. We are grateful to Keith Moore for his assistance with this collection, and to Sir Ralph Verney, Bt, for permission to quote from the Claydon letters.

The Florence Nightingale Museum in London maintains a collection of Nightingale memorabilia, as well as a collection of her books. We would like to thank Alex Attewell, Assistant Curator, for allowing us to examine this material.

We are grateful to Baruch College for granting leave during which much of the research was accomplished.

A number of individuals have assisted us in the course of our research, and we gratefully acknowledge their contributions: Robert Hayes, Periodicals Division, Brooklyn Public Library, for assisting us in the copying of the microfiche; Alicia Adams for typing the manuscript; Louisa Moy, Interlibrary Loan Division, Baruch College Library, for retrieving nineteenth- and twentieth-century monographs from across the country; Kathyrn Johnson, Assistant Professor of Historical Theology, Louisville Seminary, for her helpful suggestions; Edwin W. Macrae for reading portions of the manuscript; Mrs. Celia Winkworth of the Royal Surgical Aid Society for her hospitality at Lea Hurst, Nightingale's childhood home; and Rosie and Geneviève for their companionship.

Introduction

Many years ago, I had a large and very curious acquaintance among the artisans of the North of England and of London. I learned that they were without any religion whatever—though diligently seeking after one, principally in Comte and his school. Any return to what is called Christianity appeared impossible. It is for them this book was written.[1]

"This book," *Suggestions for Thought to the Searchers after Truth among the Artizans of England*, was an 829-page work in three volumes that Florence Nightingale had privately printed in 1860. She affectionately referred to it as her "Stuff." Her motivation for writing her "Stuff" was to offer the artisans, or working class people of England, an alternative to atheism. Disillusioned with conventional religion and weary of ungrounded metaphysical speculation, many were turning to the positivist philosophy of Auguste Comte,[2] in which all valid knowledge is based on verifiable propositions. Nightingale was also an empiricist, but, instead of abolishing the concept of God as did Comte, she sought to unify science and religion in a way that would bring order, meaning, and purpose to human life. Sir Edward Cook, Nightingale's early and still most authoritative biographer, wrote that *Suggestions for Thought* has conspicuous merits along with equally conspicuous defects:

> The merits are of the substance; the defects are of form and arrangement; but Miss Nightingale never found time or strength or inclination—I know not which or how many of the three were wanting—to remove the defects by recasting the book. Unpublished, therefore, it is likely, I suppose, to remain. But as it stands it is a remarkable work. No one, indeed, could read it without being impressed by the powerful mind, the spiritual force, and (with some qualifications) the literary ability of the writer. If she had not during her more active years been absorbed in practical affairs, or if at a later time her energy or inclination had not been impaired by ill health, Miss Nightingale might have attained a place among the philosophical writers of the nineteenth century.[3]

---

1. Letter to John Stuart Mill (Sept. 5, 1860). The correspondence between Nightingale and Mill on the subject of *Suggestions for Thought* is contained in "Florence Nightingale as a Leader in the Religious and Civic Thought of Her Time."
2. For Nightingale's views on positivism, see Chapter 2, "On Universal Law."
3. Sir Edward Cook, *Life of Florence Nightingale*, vol. 1, p. 470.

Although Nightingale was best known for her writings on nursing practice, she also wrote extensively on the subjects of nursing education and administration, hospital construction and administration, sanitation, statistics, social reform, the health of the British soldier, and the improvement of the farming systems of India. Most of her writings were in the form of privately printed reports, papers published in conference proceedings, and newspaper and journal articles.[4] The context or basis for all her work, however, is found in *Suggestions for Thought*. Although Nightingale expressed her opinions on spiritual matters in diary entries and in letters to family and friends, *Suggestions for Thought*, together with two 1873 articles in *Fraser's Magazine*,[5] are the only works exclusively devoted to the explication of her spiritual philosophy.

Nightingale, who lived for ninety years (1820–1910), wrote *Suggestions for Thought* when she was in her thirties. The work is thus a product of the young Florence Nightingale, and should be understood within the context of her intellectual and emotional life at that time. Accordingly, this introduction, rather than being a chronologically ordered biography, is a summary of some of the major influences—philosophies, persons, and events—that helped shape her thinking at an early age and thus form the background to *Suggestions for Thought*. Many of these influences are also treated in the commentary where they relate to specific issues in Nightingale's text. Significant events in Nightingale's life are listed in the Chronology at the end of this volume.

The Passionate Statistician

Named for the Italian city in which she was born, Florence was the younger of two daughters born to William Edward and Frances ("Fanny") Smith Nightingale. Both parents came from wealthy British backgrounds: her father, the heir to an estate, and her mother, the daughter of a philanthropic Member of Parliament.

William Edward Nightingale, or W.E.N., as he was called, personally supervised the education of his daughters. A graduate of Cambridge and a liberal-minded Unitarian, his views on the education of women were much in advance of his time. He taught Florence and her older sister Parthenope

4. See Bishop and Goldie, *A Bio-Bibliography of Florence Nightingale*.
5. "A 'Note' of Interrogation"; "A Sub-'Note' of Interrogation."

history, philosophy, French, Italian, German, Latin, and classical Greek. A member of the British Association for the Advancement of Science, W.E.N. took the family to its meetings and, on at least one occasion, entertained a number of the scientists at the Nightingales' estate.[6] A "commonplace" book in which Florence kept lesson notes during her adolescence indicates that her education included rudiments of chemistry, geography, physics, and astronomy.[7] Florence was much more interested in mathematics than was her father, however, and she had to pursue the subject on her own because W.E.N. was reluctant to engage an instructor.[8]

Because of Nightingale's natural predilection for collecting and analyzing data, her interest in mathematics turned into a passion for statistics. She enjoyed reading statistical tables, particularly those dealing with nursing and public health, as most people enjoy reading novels. While in the Crimea (November 1854 to July 1856) she not only cared for the wounded, served as an auxiliary purveyor, and instituted sanitary reforms, but also systematized the careless record keeping practices of the military hospitals. In a lengthy report entitled *Notes on Matters Affecting the Health, Efficiency and Hospital Administration of the British Army* (1858), she pioneered the graphical representation of statistics, illustrating with charts and diagrams how improved sanitation decreased the rate of mortality.[9] This report served as the blueprint for a large scale system of reforms introduced by her friend Sidney Herbert, the Secretary at War, during the years 1859–1861.

Nightingale was deeply influenced by the work of Lambert-Adolph-Jacques Quetelet (1796–1874), the Belgian astronomer and natural scientist who is generally regarded as the founder of modern social statistics. In 1841 Quetelet organized the Commission Central de Statistique, which became the central agency for the collection of statistics in Belgium and set the standard for similar organizations throughout Europe. His efforts to achieve international cooperation in statistics led to the founding of the International Statistical Congress in 1853. Nightingale was a member of this organization and met with Quetelet when he traveled to England in 1860.[10]

Quetelet applied the statistical method to social dynamics (most notably the yearly crime rates in various groups) illustrating regularities in human behavior. He felt, as did Nightingale, that these regularities were

6. Goldie, *A Calendar of the Letters of Florence Nightingale*, microfiche 2.A11,288.
7. BM Add. MSS. 45848.
8. Woodham-Smith, *Florence Nightingale, 1820–1910*, pp. 26–28.
9. Some of her diagrams have been reproduced in Cohen, "Florence Nightingale."
10. *Calendar of Letters*, 7.A14,345.

caused by the social conditions of these groups and that legislation which improved social conditions would also improve human behavior. Unlike many of their contemporaries, who were committed to the doctrines of free will and individual responsibility, Quetelet and Nightingale felt that human will is subject to law, as is everything else in the universe. "If we could entirely know the character and circumstances of a man," Nightingale wrote, "we might predict his future conduct with mathematical precision."[11]

Nightingale was not only a "passionate statistician,"[12] as Cook described her, but also a "reverent statistician." In her view, God is the Divine Mind who organizes the universe through scientific laws. These laws or organizing principles are discovered through the study of statistical patterns. Statistics is thus a sacred science that allows one to transcend one's narrow, individual experience and read the thoughts of God.

The Western Mystical Tradition

By the time she was in her teens, Nightingale had mastered the elements of classical Greek and had translated portions of Plato's *Phaedo*, *Crito*, and *Apology*.[13] Plato's metaphysical philosophy greatly appealed to her and influenced her view of the world. Some of the main concepts in *Suggestions for Thought*, for example, the material world as the imperfect expression of a transcendent reality, can be traced back to Plato. In her later years, she helped her friend Benjamin Jowett, the classical scholar and Master of Balliol College at Oxford, revise his translation of the *Dialogues of Plato* (published in 1875). She annotated his summaries and introductions, and at his request sent him copious suggestions for revision. He referred to her as a "first-rate Critic" who kept him up to a higher standard:

> I cannot be too grateful to you for criticizing Plato. . . . I have adopted nearly all your hints as far as I have gone (however many hints I might give you, my belief is that you would never adopt any of them).[14]

It is perhaps from the study of Plato that Nightingale became deeply interested in the Christian mystics. She mentioned to Jowett that there

---

11. *Suggestions for Thought*, vol. 1, p. 153. Unless otherwise noted, all quotations attributed to Nightingale in the introduction and commentary are from the original three volumes.
12. Cook, *Life of Florence Nightingale*, vol. 1, p. 435.
13. Cook, *Life of Florence Nightingale*, vol. 1, p. 13.
14. 30 April 1874. Quinn and Prest, *Dear Miss Nightingale*, p. 257.

were "curious analogies" between the writings of Plato and those of medieval mystics such as Francis of Assisi and John of the Cross. With great interest she read Thomas à Kempis's *The Imitation of Christ*, copiously marking and annotating her copy with personal reflections.[15] Her attraction to the mystics was, she wrote, a result of the fact that they were "not for Church but *for* God," and that they threw overboard "all that mechanism & lived for God alone."[16]

During the years 1873–74 she worked on a book of extracts from various mystical writings which was to be entitled *Notes from Devotional Authors of the Middle Ages, Collected, Chosen, and Freely Translated by Florence Nightingale*. The book was unfortunately never completed, but Sir Edward Cook was able to reconstruct the preface from her various notes and rough drafts. In the following passages, she presents her view of mysticism and the spiritual life.

> For what is Mysticism? Is it not the attempt to draw near to God, not by rites or ceremonies, but by inward disposition? Is it not merely a hard word for "The Kingdom of Heaven is within"? Heaven is neither a place nor a time. There might be a Heaven not only *here* but *now* . . .

> That Religion is not devotion, but work and suffering for love of God; this is the true doctrine of Mystics—as is more particularly set forth in a definition of the 16th century: "True religion is to have no other will but God's."

> Christ Himself was the first true Mystic. "My meat is to do the will of Him that sent me and to finish His work." What is this but putting in fervent and the most striking words the foundation of all real Mystical Religion?—which is that for all our actions, all our words, all our thoughts, the food upon which they are to live and have their being is to be the indwelling Presence of God, the union with God; that is, with the Spirit of Goodness and Wisdom.

> Where shall I find God? In myself. That is the true Mystical Doctrine. But then I myself must be in a state for Him to come and dwell in me. This is the whole aim of the Mystical Life; and all Mystical Rules in all times and countries have been laid down for putting the soul into such a state.[17]

In spite of her emphasis on Christian mysticism, Nightingale argued that "you must go to Mahometanism, to Buddhism, to the East, to the Sufis & Fakirs, to Pantheism, for the right growth of mysticism."[18] As will be

15. In the collection of the Florence Nightingale Museum, London.
16. BM Add. MSS. 47735.f226.
17. Cited in Cook, *Life of Florence Nightingale*, vol. 2, p. 233.
18. Letter dated 2 March [1853], Claydon Collection (*Calendar of Letters*, 3.C14,659).

shown subsequently, Nightingale became well versed in the spiritual traditions of the east.

Thus at the center of Nightingale's spiritual philosophy is a concept that undergirds all the mystical traditions: that the universe is the incarnation or embodiment of a transcendent God, and that human beings, through a change in consciousness, are able to experience the underlying divinity of themselves and their world.[19] In Nightingale's view, all phenomena are regulated by law, and thus mystical union with God can be knowledgeably facilitated by creating the appropriate circumstances. Society should be organized, she thought, in a way that would help each individual attain physical and spiritual health, "for putting the soul into such a state" for the indwelling of the divine life. She found conventional society, including the Church of England of which she was a nominal member, sadly lacking.

She was particularly interested in the Roman Catholic religious orders, especially those devoted to serving the poor, because they represented an attempt to organize life around a spiritual purpose. During a six-month visit to Rome when she was twenty-seven years old, she went on a ten-day retreat at the convent of the Trinità de Monte. There she met Madre Santa Colomba, who had such a profound effect on her that two years later, while traveling in Egypt, she still felt the influence of her "madre" (see below). Although she attended mass and was received by the Pope, she tried to reassure her parents that she was not converting:

> Are you afraid that I am becoming a Roman Catholic? I might perhaps, if there had been anything in me for Roman Catholicism to lay hold of, but I was not a Protestant before. . . . Can either of these two [churches] be true? Can the "word" be pinned down to either one period or one church? All churches are, of course, only more or less unsuccessful attempts to represent the unseen to the mind.[20]

Despite these remarks to her family, Nightingale was indeed tempted to convert to Roman Catholicism, because she felt it offered more opportunities for women than did the Church of England. She discussed the issue with her friend the Rev. Henry Edward Manning,[21] a recent convert to Catholicism, who was working with the poor in the East End of London:

19. Aldous Huxley, *The Perennial Philosophy*. This work is an anthology such as Nightingale had planned to organize, but broader because it contains excerpts from a number of writings of eastern mystics that were not readily available in Nightingale's time.

20. Quoted in Keele, ed., *Florence Nightingale in Rome: Letters Written by Florence Nightingale in Rome in the Winter of 1847–1848*, p. 155.

21. He later became the famous Cardinal Manning, whose biography, as well as Florence

But you do know now, with all its faults, what a home the Catholic Church is. And yet what is she to you compared with what she would be to me? No one can tell, no man can tell what she is to women—their training, their discipline, their hope, their home—to women because they are left wholly uneducated by the Church of England, almost wholly uncared-for—while men are not. For what training is there compared to that of the Catholic nun?...There is nothing like the training (in these days) which the Sacred Heart or the Order of St. Vincent gives to women.[22]

In the summer of 1852, while Nightingale was considering converting to Roman Catholicism, she was also preparing a 65-page proof of *Suggestions for Thought*. The content of the proof (much of which was included in the expanded work) centered on the lawful universe, a concept inconsistent with many widely held beliefs, such as God's forgiveness of sins, Christ's atonement, and the verity of miracles as recorded in the Bible. After reading her work, Manning prudently advised her *not* to convert as her views were far too radical. Although it would appear contradictory of Nightingale to consider converting to a church which "insists peremptorily upon my believing what I cannot believe,"[23] it illustrates her deep need to be part of an organization or institution through which she could channel her talent and energy, and which would help her give outward form to her inner life.

The Founder of Modern Nursing

It was somewhat of an exaggeration for Nightingale to write that the Church of England left women "almost wholly uncared-for." The Anglo-Catholic revival represented by Tractarianism (see commentary in Chapter 1, "On the Concept of God") in the 1840s had stimulated the growth of women's religious orders modeled on Roman Catholic sisterhoods.[24] Edward Bouverie Pusey (1800–1882), the High Church reformer, influenced the founding of the Sisterhood of the Holy Cross in 1845, and his friend

Nightingale's, is included in Strachey's *Eminent Victorians*. See also Robert Gray, *Cardinal Manning: A Biography*.

22. Letter to Henry Manning, 15 July 1852. Vicinus and Nergaard, *Ever Yours, Florence Nightingale: Selected Letters*, p. 59. Ellipsis in original. The Order of St. Vincent is discussed below, pp. 92, 142; the Sacred Heart community cannot be identified with certainty.

23. Letter to Henry Manning, 15 July 1852.

24. A discussion of the economic and social factors associated with the revival of the non-Catholic sisterhoods can be found in Anne Summer, "Ministering Angels." See also A. M. Allchin, *The Silent Rebellion: Anglican Religious Communities, 1845–1900*; Michael Hill, *The Religious Order: A Study of Virtuoso Religion and Its Legitimation in the Nineteenth-Century Church of England*; and Gail Malmgreen, ed., *Religion in the Lives of English Women: 1760–1930*.

Priscilla Lydia Sellon established the Sisterhood of Mercy of Devonport and Plymouth in 1848. The first nursing sisterhood of the Church of England, the Training Institution for Nurses, St. John's House, was also founded in 1848. Nightingale showed little interest in these groups, and did not refer to them in *Suggestions for Thought*. The reasons for her lack of interest are unclear, but she did not support the Tractarian movement with which the Anglican sisterhoods were affiliated, and this position likely influenced her opinion of the sisterhoods themselves.

Nightingale spent a short time at the hospital of the Sisters of Charity in Paris in 1853 and three months at the Institution for Deaconesses at Kaiserswerth, Germany in 1851. The Institution had been founded in 1833 by Theodore Fliedner (1800–1864), an Evangelical pastor and philanthropist, and his wife as a refuge for women recently discharged from prison, but grew to include a hospital, nursery school, and orphanage. Years after her apprenticeship at Kaiserswerth, Nightingale wrote: ". . . never have I met with a higher tone, a purer devotion than there. There was no neglect." And yet: "the hospital was certainly the worst part of Kaiserswerth. I took all the training that was to be had—there was none to be had in England, but Kaiserswerth was far from having trained me."[25]

Nightingale was thus largely self-taught in the area of nursing. For years, she got up before dawn to study hospital and public health reports, making her own statistical analyses; she inspected hospitals all over England and abroad; and she took every opportunity to care personally for the ill, both within her own extended family and among the poor in the villages near her country estate. Nightingale acquired her nursing knowledge (that is, "knowledge of the laws of health") through observation and experience. Health is not an arbitrary gift of God, she concluded, but a state human beings must achieve for themselves. "With regard to health or sickness," she wrote in *Suggestions for Thought*, "these are not 'sent' to try us, but are the results of keeping, or not keeping, the laws of God; and, therefore, it would be 'conformable to the will of God' to keep His laws, so that you *would* have health."[26]

Her classic text, *Notes on Nursing* (1860), can be viewed as a practical application of the central concepts in *Suggestions for Thought*. Healing, like all physical phenomena, is a lawful process. It is regulated by nature, that is, the expression or manifestation of God. Through careful observation,

25. Quoted in Cook, *Life of Florence Nightingale*, vol. 1, pp. 111, 113; see also Vicinus and Nergaard, *Ever Yours, Florence Nightingale*, pp. 53, 433.
26. *Suggestions for Thought*, vol. 2, p. 119.

nursing must discover the laws of healing, such as the need for proper nourishment, ventilation, cleanliness, and quiet, and thus be able to cooperate consciously in the restorative process. "Nature alone cures," she wrote, "and what nursing has to do . . . is to put the patient in the best condition for nature to act upon him."[27]

Unfortunately, at the time of the Crimean War (1853–56), not only were "the very elements of nursing . . . all but unknown,"[28] but secular hospital nursing was considered menial work for which little training was required. Nurses were often recruited from the ranks of street women, among whom alcoholism and sexual promiscuity were common. Charles Dickens caricaturized the nurse of the day in his portrayal of Sairey Gamp in *Martin Chuzzlewit*. Because hospital nursing had such a bad reputation, most parents (including the Nightingales) were horrified if their daughters evinced an interest in this type of work, and thus nursing lost a great many intelligent and compassionate women. Indeed, when Nightingale was asked by the government to select a group of nurses to work in the military hospitals in the Crimea, she had a difficult time finding qualified applicants.[29] It was not only to help relieve the suffering of the soldiers, therefore, that she accepted this challenge:

> The consideration of overwhelming importance was the opportunity offered to advance the cause of nursing. Were nurses capable of being employed with success to nurse men under such conditions? The eyes of the nation were fixed upon Scutari. If the nurses acquitted themselves creditably, never again would they be despised. "If this succeeds," Sidney Herbert had written, "an enormous amount of good will have been done now...a prejudice will have been broken through and a precedent established which will multiply the good to all time."[30]

Toward the end of the war, a Nightingale Fund was established as a thank offering from the people of England. The fund was used to establish the first non-sectarian nursing school, the Nightingale Training School at St. Thomas's Hospital in London.

---

27. *Notes on Nursing: What It Is, and What It Is Not*, p. 133.

28. *Notes on Nursing*, p. 8.

29. Of the original group of thirty-eight, ten were Roman Catholic nuns; fourteen were Anglican Sisters (eight from Miss Sellon's sisterhood and six from St. John's House); the remainder were from various hospitals.

30. 15 October, 1854, quoted in Cook, *Life of Florence Nightingale*, vol. 1, p. 153. Ellipsis in original.

The Struggle for Fulfillment

For Nightingale, service to God is service to Humanity. Mystical union with God is not an end in itself, but the source of strength and guidance for doing one's work in the world. The aim of human life, she wrote, is to create heaven—here and now—on the earth: "The 'kingdom of heaven is within,' indeed, but we must also create one without, because we are *intended* to act upon our circumstances."[31]

Unfortunately, however, Nightingale's sense of vocation created a great deal of friction in her family life. Bored and frustrated by the leisured life of an upper class young woman, Florence wrote: "I craved for some regular occupation, for something worth doing instead of frittering time away on useless trifles."[32] Fanny Nightingale had high social expectations for her attractive and charming daughter, and a bitter conflict arose when Florence insisted on devoting her life to nursing.

W.E.N., with his liberal views, was inclined to let Florence have her way; his character was less forceful than his wife's, however, and in the end he chose the path of least resistance. It was only after years of struggle, disappointment, and unhappiness for all concerned that Florence was given permission to study nursing at the hospital of the Sisters of Charity and at the Institution for Deaconesses in Kaiserswerth.

The frustration Nightingale felt over the lack of opportunity for women is partly responsible for the tone of discontent that pervades much of *Suggestions for Thought*. Harsh criticisms of conventional society are found throughout the second volume of her work. "There appears to be now no relation to God in anything we do," she wrote, "no reference to Him in any of our modes of life. Among the rich the reference is to how much of material enjoyment they can crowd in; among the poor, how not to starve."[33] The structure of family life came under her attack, particularly with respect to the role and position of daughters. She was infuriated by the assumption that an unmarried woman would stay at home, cater to the whims of the family, and follow her own interests at "odd moments."

> The maxim of doing things at "odd moments" is a most dangerous one. Would not a painter spoil his picture by working on it "at odd moments?" If it be a

31. *Suggestions for Thought*, vol. 2, p. 205.
32. Quoted in Woodham-Smith, *Florence Nightingale, 1820–1910*, p. 9. This biography details the family conflict over Florence's choice of a career.
33. *Suggestions for Thought*, vol. 2, p. 105.

picture worth painting at all, and if he be a man of genius, he must have the whole of his picture in his head every time he touches it, and this requires great concentration, and this concentration cannot be obtained at "odd moments," and if he works without it he will spoil his work. Can we fancy Michael Angelo running up and putting on a touch to his Sistine ceiling at "odd moments"?[34]

John Stuart Mill, one of the few people who received a copy of *Suggestions for Thought* when it was first printed in 1860, was particularly struck by Nightingale's social criticisms. In *The Subjection of Women*, written in 1861 and published in 1869, Mill directly alluded to her work:

> . . . if he [a man] has a pursuit, he offends nobody by devoting his time to it; occupation is received as a valid excuse for his not answering to every casual demand which may be made on him. Are a woman's occupations, especially her chosen and voluntary ones, ever regarded as excusing her from any of what are termed the calls of society? . . . She must always be at the beck and call of somebody, generally of everybody. If she has a study or a pursuit, she must snatch any short interval which accidently occurs to be employed in it. *A celebrated woman, in a work which I hope will some day be published, remarks truly that everything a woman does is done at odd times.* Is it wonderful, then, if she does not attain the highest eminence in things which require consecutive attention, and the concentration on them of the chief interest of life?[35]

Years later, Virginia Woolf referred to these same social criticisms of Nightingale's in *A Room of One's Own* (1929), her classic book about women and fiction:

> If a woman wrote, she would have to write in the common sitting-room. And, as Miss Nightingale was so vehemently to complain,—"women never have an half hour . . . that they can call their own"—she was always interrupted. Still it would be easier to write prose and fiction there than to write poetry or a play. Less concentration is required. Jane Austen wrote like that to the end of her days.[36]

Woolf's footnote indicates that the quotation was taken from "Cassandra," an essay (or "novel" as Nightingale called it) on the confined life of a woman in upper class British society. Nightingale had written the essay in 1852 and then appended it to the second volume of *Suggestions for Thought*. "Cassandra" was published separately in 1928 as an appendix to Ray

---

34. *Suggestions for Thought*, vol. 2, pp. 65–66.
35. John Stuart Mill, *The Subjection of Women*, p. 75. Emphasis added.
36. Virginia Woolf, *A Room of One's Own*, pp. 69–70.

Strachey's *The Cause: A Short History of the Women's Movement in Great Britain*;[37] Woolf indicated that it was Strachey's edition from which she was working. It is evident that Nightingale's words were on Woolf's mind when she was writing *A Room of One's Own*. She referred to Nightingale several times and many of her ideas are similar to those in "Cassandra" and other sections of *Suggestions for Thought*: the importance of one's state of mind for creative work; the necessity of money, time, and privacy for achieving that state of mind; and the creative process as an evolutionary phenomenon unfolding throughout history.

Suggestions for Thought is an excellent illustration of Virginia Woolf's thesis in *A Room of One's Own*. Tracing the history of women and fiction, she observes that, with a few notable exceptions such as Jane Austen, who had in some way made peace with the narrowness of her circumstances, the artistry of women's work has been distorted by bitterness and frustration:

> The reason perhaps why we know so little of Shakespeare . . . is that his grudges and spites and antipathies are hidden from us. We are not held up by some "revelation" which reminds us of the writer. All desire to protest, to preach, to proclaim an injury, to pay off a score, to make the world the witness of some hardship or grievance was fired out of him and consumed. Therefore his poetry flows from him free and unimpeded. If ever a human being got his work expressed completely, it was Shakespeare. If ever a mind was incandescent, unimpeded . . . it was Shakespeare's mind . . .
> . . . and when people compare Shakespeare and Jane Austen they may mean that the minds of both had consumed all impediments; and for that reason we do not know Jane Austen and we do not know Shakespeare, and for that reason Jane Austen pervades every word that she wrote, and so does Shakespeare.[38]

Unfortunately, Nightingale's mind, with all its greatness, was not "incandescent." As Woolf comments, "Florence Nightingale shrieked aloud in her agony."[39] Scathing criticisms of the "prison" of family life in which the daughters are being "murdered" erupt into the second volume of *Suggestions for Thought*, taking the reader by surprise and disrupting the flow of the philosophical discussion. To strengthen the integrity of the work, we had planned to organize this material into an appendix, but later decided to give it a chapter of its own within the text. This is truer to the

37. "Cassandra" was later published as a separate volume by the Feminist Press (1980), and again in Mary Poovey's *Cassandra and Suggestions for Thought* (1990).
38. *A Room of One's Own*, pp. 58, 71.
39. *A Room of One's Own*, pp. 57–58.

original work and also to Florence Nightingale herself, for the painful struggle to achieve fulfillment as a brilliant woman in nineteenth-century England was, indeed, an integral part of her life.

Unitarianism

Because Nightingale had been raised in the Anglican church and was deeply attracted to the religious orders of the Roman Catholic church, it comes as no surprise that most of her comments on organized religion in *Suggestions for Thought* focus on these two churches. It has been noted previously, however, that she may also have been influenced by Unitarian ideas because both parents came from Unitarian backgrounds. (Fanny Nightingale chose to rear her daughters in the Church of England probably for reasons of prestige.[40]) Nightingale's maternal grandfather, William Smith (1756–1835), was a prominent Unitarian Member of Parliament dedicated to securing rights for "dissenters" (non-Anglican Protestants) as well as Catholics. Smith convinced Parliament in 1813 to pass the Unitarian Toleration Act, which made denying the divinity of Christ no longer a crime.[41] Smith was also a supporter of Joseph Priestley (1733–1804), an outspoken Unitarian theologian and scientist (he discovered oxygen) whose radical opinions on religion and politics incited a riot in 1791, compelling him to flee to America. Nightingale recorded in a letter (ca. 1840) that her Uncle Sam (Samuel Smith, her mother's brother) read Dr. Priestley to the family.[42] That Nightingale was familiar with Priestley's work is also evident from her remarks in *Suggestions for Thought* (see Chapter 7, "On Life After Death").

Unitarians were distinguished by their rejection of the Trinity and of the divinity of Christ. They also disputed such beliefs as original sin, predestination, the atonement, the last judgement, and eternal damnation. Although initially Unitarians based their beliefs on scripture, under the growing influence of German biblical criticism (see below) and the leadership of James Martineau (1805–1900),[43] a more liberal faction developed

40. Widerquist, "The Spirituality of Florence Nightingale."

41. Edwards, *Christian England*, vol. 3, *From the 18th Century to the First World War*, p. 111. See Also "Smith, William" entry in the *Dictionary of National Biography*.

42. *Calendar of Letters*, 1.D14,120. Priestley's writings include the two-volume *General History of the Christian Church to the Fall of the Western Empire*.

43. James Martineau upheld the theist position (see below) against the negations of the physical sciences. He was the brother of the writer and anti-slavery advocate Harriet Martineau (1802–76), with whom Nightingale corresponded for many years. Nightingale records

whose adherents looked for solace in human reason and conscience rather than in the scriptures or church. Social causes such as prison reform, education, temperance, and women's rights became increasingly central to the work of the Unitarian community.

Although Nightingale held many beliefs in common with Unitarians, and like them was concerned with "deeds not creeds," if we can judge from the few remarks in *Suggestions for Thought*, Unitarianism on the whole does not seem to have impressed her. She referred to it as "dull" because, like Judaism, it was "pure Monotheism," and noted that while Unitarians had eliminated Christ and the Holy Ghost as objects of worship they had not succeeded in making God "more loved or more loveable."[44] She clearly spoke in terms of the Trinity (see Chapter 6, "On the Spiritual Life"), and believed that all people, like Christ, are "incarnations of God" (see Chapter 1, "On the Concept of God")—ideas that are contrary to Unitarian beliefs.

The Influence from Germany and the East

Because dissenters were barred from attending Oxford and Cambridge Universities until 1854 and 1856 respectively, many Unitarians went abroad to study and thereby became familiar with German theology, which had a decidedly liberal bent. By the nineteenth century, Germany was far more advanced than England in the areas of theology, biblical criticism, and historical scholarship. At the end of the previous century, the German theologian Friedrich Schleiermacher (1768–1834) had addressed his remarks in *Religion: Speeches to Its Cultured Despisers* (1799) to the "sons of Germany," maintaining that they alone were capable and worthy of having awakened "the sense for holy and divine things," while the English knew "nothing of religion."[45] This sentiment was later corroborated in England by Mark Pattison, rector of Lincoln College, who noted that "It is now in Germany alone that the vital questions of Religion are discussed with the full and free application of all the resources of learning and criticism which our age has at its command."[46] This development can perhaps be traced

---

in a letter (ca. 1853) that her Aunt Mai went to hear James Martineau preach (*Calendar of Letters*, 3.D5,677).

44. *Suggestions for Thought*, vol. 2, p. 308.

45. *Religion: Speeches to Its Cultured Despisers* (1958 ed.), p. 9.

46. Pattison, "Present State of Theology in Germany." Mark Pattison (1813–1884), rector of Lincoln College, was raised an Evangelical and was later influenced by J. H. Newman and Pusey; he came to hold liberal opinions on religion, however, becoming a Broad Churchman and contributing to *Essays and Reviews*.

back to the reign of Frederick II, the "Great" (1712–86), King of Prussia (1740–1786), who advocated religious toleration among his subjects. Although a number of socio-political factors contributed to religious unrest in the Victorian Church, the influence of German scholarship on English freethinkers should not be underestimated. Writers Samuel Coleridge and Thomas Carlyle did much to introduce German intellectualism into England, as did George Eliot,[47] who in 1846 undertook a translation of David Friedrich Strauss's *Das Leben Jesu*. Strauss's highly controversial work (with which Nightingale was familiar[48]) argued for a mythological interpretation of the New Testament, thereby denying the divinity of Jesus, his incarnation, miracles, and resurrection.

By age twenty, Florence Nightingale too was studying German, and reading the works of the German orientalist and theologian Heinrich Ewald (1803–1875).[49] In a letter to her parents from Paris in 1853, Nightingale listed "German Metaphysics" among her principal reading interests (along with "Catholic Rules" and the French philosophers Auguste Comte and Victor Cousin),[50] and she herself noted on several occasions that Germany was more advanced than England in terms of religion and philosophy.[51] She had ample opportunity to explore German scholarship through her friendships with the German orientalists Julius von Mohl (1800–1876) and Christian Carl Josias von Bunsen (1791–1860). Through her friendships with these men, the young Florence Nightingale became familiar with the works of leading German theologians and historians, and became conversant in the spiritual legacy of the Near and Far East. This is evidenced by her letters and personal notes, which contain discussions of ancient Egyptian religion, Islam, Zoroastrianism, Hinduism, and Buddhism.[52]

Known primarily for his translation of the Persian epic *Shah Nameh* ("Book of Kings") by Firdausi, Julius von Mohl was the husband of Mary Clarke, a close friend of Nightingale's, whose home in Paris was a popular

47. George Eliot was an acquaintance of Nightingale's and had many friends in common with her, including Benjamin Jowett, J. A. Froude, Max Müller, and Frederick Denison Maurice (see below). Eliot wrote of Nightingale: "There is a loftiness of mind about her which is well expressed by her form and manner" (*Life of George Eliot as Related in Her Letters and Journals*, p. 145).

48. BM Add. MSS. 45845.f25.

49. *Calendar of Letters*, 1.E1,124ff; 2.E6,433. Ewald also authored a Hebrew grammar Nightingale may have used in her studies of that language (2.F14,502).

50. *Calendar of Letters*, 3.E3,717

51. *Calendar of Letters*, 3.D11,697; 17.C4,87.

52. BM Add. MSS. 45845.f137; 45793.f75; letter to Parthenope, 10 March [1853]; letter to her parents, [Paris, 1853], Claydon Collection (*Calendar of Letters*, 3.C14,659; 3.D9,692).

gathering place of intellectuals. Nightingale corresponded with Mohl on politics, literature, philosophy, and religion, and on several occasions pressed him for his opinion on gnosticism,[53] a religious and philosophical movement of the Hellenistic and early Christian world that combined elements from Judaism, Christianity, and other sources and emphasized secret knowledge. She was probably interested in the Gnostics because, like her, they sought spiritual truth through their own inner development rather than through the intercession of the Church. According to Cook, Mohl had great admiration for Nightingale's intellect, and she "regarded his studies in eastern religion as a real contribution to 'theodike,' one of her principal preoccupations."[54] Nightingale's confidence in Mohl's intellectual abilities was such that she considered him the ideal person to edit *Suggestions for Thought*.[55]

The German diplomat and scholar Christian Carl Josias von Bunsen, Prussian ambassador to the Court of St. James from 1842 to 1854, also proved to be of considerable importance to Florence Nightingale's intellectual and spiritual development. Nightingale frequented Bunsen's home in London, which had become a center of scholarly activity, and sought his advice on matters of both a personal and academic nature. He introduced her to the works of the great German philosophers, historians, and theologians of the day, such as Arthur Schopenhauer (1788–1860), Barthold Niebuhr (see below), and Friedrich Schleiermacher,[56] as well as the prominent English intellectuals and clergymen who comprised the "Broad Church" movement (see below). By means of her association with Bunsen and his colleagues, Nightingale was exposed to the spiritual traditions of the East as well as to elements of heterodox theology seen clearly in *Suggestions for Thought*.

The Baroness Bunsen indicates that the friendship between Nightingale and her husband commenced in 1842, when Florence was twenty-two years of age, and that he

> from the first valued her, on a few occasions, when nothing occurred peculiarly to rouse and reveal the soul which subsisted in her, in the fullness of its energy,

53. BM Add. MSS. 46385.ff15–17.

54. Cook, *Life of Florence Nightingale*, vol. 2, p. 317. *Theodike* or theodicy, a term coined by the philosopher Gottfried Liebniz (1646–1716), is a compound of the Greek words for God (*theos*) and justice (*dike*), and refers to the attempt to reconcile the benevolence, omnipotence, and justice of God with the existence of evil. Nightingale's theodicy is explicated in Chapter 4, "On Sin and Evil."

55. BM Add. MSS. 45790.f248.

56. Schleiermacher published translations of Plato; Platonic philosophy was crucial to the development of his spiritual views as for Nightingale's.

or the powers which only waited for an opportunity to be developed; but her calm dignity of deportment, self-conscious without either shyness or presumption, and the few words indicating deep reflection, just views, and clear perceptions of life and its obligations, and the trifling acts showing forgetfulness of self and devotedness to others, were of sufficient force to bring conviction to the observer, even before it had been proved by all outward experience, that she was possessed of all that moral greatness which her subsequent course of action, suffering, and of influential power, has displayed.[57]

Bunsen's significance goes much beyond his personal influence on Nightingale and her work, however, for, as R. A. D. Owen wrote in his study of Bunsen, "Certainly few men of foreign birth ever played so prominent a part in the religious discussions of the nation [i.e., England], certainly, none in the nineteenth century."[58]

Despite his career as a diplomat, Bunsen was primarily a scholar of ancient and oriental languages and mythology, as well as a theologian.[59] In addition to Latin, Greek, and Hebrew, Bunsen studied ancient Egyptian, Chinese, Persian, and Arabic, and for some time considered a journey to India to perform linguistic research. He described his scholarly objectives as follows:

I remain firm, and strive after my earliest purpose in life, more felt, perhaps, than already discerned,—namely, to bring over into my own knowledge and into my own Fatherland the language and the spirit of the solemn and distant East. I would for the accomplishment of this object even quit Europe, in order to draw out of the ancient well that which I found not elsewhere.[60]

Bunsen applied his philological and historical knowledge to the study of scripture as means of enhancing religion—not threatening it as conservatives feared. He studied Jewish, Christian, Islamic, and Hindu scriptures, and the works of authors as diverse as the "heretic" Giordano Bruno (see below) and the Persian mystic Jalal ud-Din Rumi.[61] Like Nightingale, he was interested in the works of Plato and the Christian mystics.

In 1817, Bunsen entered diplomatic service in Rome under the tutelage of his mentor Barthold Niebuhr (1776–1831), a noted historian and the Prussian ambassador to the Vatican, whom he succeeded as Counsellor of

57. *Memoirs of Baron Bunsen*, vol. 2, pp. 12–13.

58. R. A. D. Owen, *Christian Bunsen and Liberal English Theology*, p. 83.

59. English translations of his works include *The Church of the Future* (1847), *Egypt's Place in Universal History* (5 vols., 1848–60), *Hippolytus and His Age* (2 vols., 1852), *Christianity and Mankind* (7 vols., 1854), *Signs of the Times* (1856), and *God in History* (3 vols., 1868–70).

60. Quoted by F. Max Müller in *Chips from a German Workshop*, vol. 3, p. 349.

61. Jalal ud-Din Rumi (1207–73) was a Sufi poet best known for his poetic exposition of Sufism, the *Mathnawi*.

the Legation in 1823. While in Rome, Bunsen formed enduring friendships with English intellectuals such as Connop Thirlwall, Julius Charles Hare, and Thomas Arnold,[62] all of whom were later subjected to criticism by religious authorities in England on account of their unorthodox views. Their interest in German scholarship in history and theology, such as Niebuhr's *History of Rome* and Schleiermacher's essay on St. Luke, which contradicted Church teachings on the chronology and origin of Scripture, provided the foundation for the "Broad Church" movement in England,[63] which will be discussed subsequently in relation to Nightingale's work. During his years in Rome, Bunsen also made the acquaintance of Richard Monckton Milnes, a student of Connop Thirlwall's who was later to become a serious contender for the hand of Florence Nightingale.[64]

Bunsen's activities were not confined to the scholarly, but extended to humanitarian endeavors. In Rome he established a Protestant infirmary where people of that faith could receive medical care without being subjected to Catholic proselytizing. Later he would also establish a hospital in London to serve the large German-speaking population there. This facility proved to be of great benefit to all community residents regardless of nationality. Bunsen's work with hospitals undoubtedly influenced Nightingale, who for a short time before going to the Crimea (1853–54) served as superintendent of the Institution for the Care of Sick Gentlewomen in Distressed Circumstances. There she worked to secularize the institution, in order that women of all faiths might be admitted and their clergymen free to attend them. Prior to Nightingale's appointment, only Anglican patients and their priests were admitted to the facilities.

Bunsen left his diplomatic post in Rome in 1838 and served briefly as envoy to the Swiss Republic from 1839–40, during which time he befriended another controversial British theologian, Frederick Denison Maurice. (Some years later Maurice would be dismissed from his position at King's College on account of his *Theological Essays*, in which he argued against the doctrine of eternal damnation, as would Nightingale in *Suggestions for Thought*.)

In 1841 Bunsen was appointed envoy to England, and met the young

62. Connop Thirlwall (1797–1875), classical historian and bishop (St. David's, Wales); Julius Charles Hare (1795–1855), archdeacon of Lewes; Thomas Arnold (1795–1842), educator and historian, headmaster at Rugby (1828–1842), father of the poet Matthew Arnold.

63. R. A. D. Owen, *Christian Bunsen and Liberal English Theology*; Robert Preyer, "Bunsen and the Anglo-American Literary Community in Rome."

64. Richard Moncton Milnes (1809–85), 1st Baron Houghton, was a poet and an active member of Parliament. He met Nightingale in 1842 and proposed marriage, but after a courtship of several years she refused him. They nevertheless remained lifelong friends and he became a trustee of the Nightingale Fund.

Florence Nightingale the following year. In addition to her intellectual interests, Nightingale sought out Bunsen's advice on matters of spirituality, asking of him, "What can an individual do, towards lifting the load of suffering from the helpless and the miserable?"[65] She was to find the answer to her query in the Institution of Deaconesses at Kaiserswerth. Bunsen was familiar with the Institution because he had gone there himself in 1844 to find qualified nurses for the German Hospital in London. Nightingale mentioned in a letter that, finding it to be "an admirable institution," he considered sending one of his daughters there.[66] Shortly after Bunsen sent Nightingale the Institution's yearbook in 1846, she noted: "There is my home, there are my brothers and sisters all at work. There my heart is and there, I trust, will one day be my body."[67]

Before leaving on an extended voyage to Egypt in November 1849, Nightingale visited with Bunsen, who provided her with the "*dernier mot* on Egyptology*," according to Nightingale's sister Parthenope.[68] Her trip to Egypt proved to be something of a spiritual catharsis as she struggled to realize her ambitions. Beginning in February 1850, she made frequent references in her diary to God calling or speaking to her. On several occasions God revealed His will to her in the words of her "madre," Santa Columba of the Convent Trinità de Monti in Rome. In early March she wrote that she had "settled the question with God,"—undoubtedly referring to her decision to dedicate her life to nursing.[69] Within a month after leaving Egypt, on her thirtieth birthday (May 12), she noted:

> To day I am 30—the age Xt began his Mission. Now no more childish things, no more vain things, no more love, no more marriage. Now Lord, let me only think of Thy will, what Thou willest me to do. O, Lord, Thy will, Thy will.[70]

Before returning to England in August 1850, she visited the hospital at Kaiserswerth, returning the following year for a three month sojourn.

The letters she wrote to her family from Egypt are also indicative of her spiritual state and contain remarkable discussions of religion, both ancient

65. Frances Baroness Bunsen, *Memoirs of Baron Bunsen*, vol. 2, p. 13.

66. Letter to Fanny Nightingale from Kaiserswerth, 16 July 1851. Quoted in Vicinus and Nergaard, *Ever Yours, Florence Nightingale*, p. 52. This is perhaps this same daughter, Frances, who prepared the German translation of Nightingale's *Notes on Nursing*; cf. Bishop and Goldie, *Bio-Bibliography of Florence Nightingale*, p. 20; *Calendar of Letters*, 6.G12,293.

67. Private note, 7 October 1846; quoted in Woodham-Smith, *Florence Nightingale*, p. 44.

68. Quoted by Anthony Sattin in Florence Nightingale's *Letters from Egypt: A Journey on the Nile, 1849–1850*, p. 12.

69. BM Add. MSS. 45846.

70. BM Add. MSS. 45846.

and modern. Her comments on ancient Egyptian religion are noteworthy because Egyptian hieroglyphs had only been deciphered as recently as 1822 by the French Egyptologist Jean François Champollion (1790–1832), a friend of Bunsen's. As evidenced by these letters from Egypt, Nightingale was familiar with hermetic writings.[71] The term "hermetic" is used to designate a body of Latin and Greek texts dating from the second and third centuries A.D. Esoteric in content and character, they are attributed to Hermes Trismegistus, the Greek counterpart of Thoth, the Egyptian god of wisdom, called "the thrice great." Although Platonic and Stoic influences are conspicuous in these writings, the texts also seem to incorporate elements of Egyptian theology. A central theme of the *Hermetica* is the emphasis on the acquisition of divine knowledge as the means for achieving an ultimate union with or absorption in God.[72] Undoubtedly Nightingale would have been attracted to this mystical component. During the Renaissance hermetic writings became known to the west primarily through the works of the philosophers Marsilio Ficino (1433–99) and Giordano Bruno. Burned as a heretic in part for espousing the virtues of ancient Egyptian occultism as related in the Hermetica, Bruno was of particular interest to Bunsen[73] and may have also influenced Nightingale's spiritual philosophy (see Chapter 4, "On Sin and Evil").

Many of the issues Nightingale would subsequently address in *Suggestions for Thought*, such as the benevolent nature of God and universal law, are discussed in her letters from Egypt in 1849–50. Universal Law, as an expression of Divine Will, occupies a prominent place in the personal philosophies of both Bunsen and Nightingale. Bunsen wrote that "whatever emanates from the spirit is a revelation of the Divine, unfolding itself according to eternal laws."[74] Later, Nightingale would speak of an "All-Ordering Power" whose thoughts are manifest as law, so that "everything, down to the minutest particular, is so governed, 'by laws which can be seen in their effects,' that not the most trifling action or feeling is left to chance . . ."[75]

---

71. The original edition of Nightingale's *Letters from Egypt*, which Parthenope had privately printed in 1854, contains more references to hermetic philosophy than does Anthony Sattin's edition.

72. Walter Scott, *Hermetica: The Ancient Greek and Latin Writings Which Contain Religious or Philosophic Teachings Ascribed to Hermes Trismegistus.*

73. In 1850, the year of Nightingale's Egyptian voyage, Bunsen wrote: "I too have studied Giordano Bruno in late years with peculiar interest and deep sympathy" (*Memoirs of Baron Bunsen*, vol. 2, p. 169).

74. Frances Baroness Bunsen, *Christian Carl Josias freiherr von Bunsen aus seinem Briefen und nach eigener Erinnerung geschildert*, von seiner Witwe, vol. I, p. 81. Translation by the present editors; the passage is not included in the English translation of the *Memoirs*.

75. "A Sub-'Note' of Interrogation," p. 25.

Despite the fact that Bunsen's historical and philological investigations had revealed inaccuracies in the literal interpretation of scripture, he, as did Nightingale, nonetheless believed that Christianity provided a moral framework for life. In a letter to the Sanskrit scholar Friedrich Max Müller (see below), Bunsen commented on the gospels and the works of the German mystic Meister Eckhart (c.1260–c.1328):

> I am delighted that you are absorbed in Eckart [sic] . . . there is nothing better, except for the Gospel of St. John. For there stands still more clearly than in the other gospel writings, that the object of life in this world is to *found the Kingdom of God on earth* . . .[76]

Nightingale too communicated this idea in her work, writing: "The 'Kingdom of heaven is within,' but we must also make it *without*."[77] She was also greatly influenced by the Gospel of John, and wrote: "For myself the mystical or spiritual religion as laid down by St. John's Gospel, however imperfectly I have lived up to it, was and is enough."[78]

As will become apparent, the spiritual philosophy espoused by Florence Nightingale in *Suggestions for Thought* contains elements not typical of either Anglican or Unitarian thought of her day, notably the evolution of consciousness, in which the individual progressively realizes his or her unity with the Divine. This concept can be found in Eckhart and Bruno, and is consistent with the writings of Teresa of Avila, with which Nightingale was familiar, but it became popular in nineteenth-century western thought primarily through the discovery of the far-eastern spiritual traditions and the study of Sanskrit and comparative religion.

In addition to her associations with Mohl and Bunsen, Nightingale may have become familiar with the fundamentals of the eastern spiritual tradition through the works of Friedrich Max Müller (1823–1900) and Rowland Williams (1817–1870).

Friedrich Max Müller, a German student of Sanskrit who was to become one of the most renowned scholars of Indian languages and literatures, came to London in 1846 to consult manuscripts in the library of the East India Company. Bunsen promptly befriended the young scholar, assisting him financially and professionally. It was Bunsen who persuaded the East India Company to publish Müller's translation of the *Rigveda*

---

76. F. Max Müller, *Chips from a German Workshop*, vol. 3, p. 487.
77. "A Sub-'Note' of Interrogation," p. 32.
78. Letter to Benjamin Jowett, 1899. Quoted in Cook, *Life of Florence Nightingale*, vol. 2, p. 366.

(1849), pointing out that "it would be a disgrace if some other country than England published this edition of the Sacred Books of the Brahmans."[79]

Although Nightingale would not meet Müller until late in life, it is likely that she was familiar with his work through Bunsen and other friends they had in common, such as Julius and Mary von Mohl.[80] Bunsen introduced Müller to the scholarly community at Oxford, where he would eventually become Professor of Comparative Philology. At Oxford, Müller met and became friends with Benjamin Jowett, the classical scholar and liberal theologian who would later figure largely in Nightingale's life, and James Anthony Froude (1818–1894), a controversial historian and novelist. When Froude was forced to resign his fellowship at Exeter College over his *Nemesis of Faith* (1849),[81] Bunsen secured for him a position in Germany, which he nevertheless declined. More than ten years after the private printing of *Suggestions for Thought*, Nightingale sent a copy of the manuscript to Froude, whose opinion was unfavorable due to its "want of focus and form." As editor of *Fraser's Magazine*, Froude did publish two of her articles in May and June 1873, "A 'Note' of Interrogation" and "A Sub-'Note' of Interrogation." Written with the encouragement of Benjamin Jowett, the articles reiterate some of the issues developed at length in *Suggestions For Thought*. The articles were widely noticed and brought her many letters, both supportive and critical. Some individuals, shocked at her views, told Nightingale that they would pray daily for her conversion!

In the late 1850s, while revising and expanding her draft of *Suggestions for Thought*, it is possible that Nightingale became familiar with a comparative study of Christianity and Hinduism by Rowland Williams entitled *A Dialogue of the Knowledge of the Supreme Lord, in Which are Compared the Claims of Christianity and Hinduism*. On reading the book, Bunsen lauded Williams as "one of the deepest scholars and philosophical minds of the age."[82] Addressing both Buddhist and Hindu systems of belief, Williams discusses concepts such as the unity of mankind, the one supreme soul

79. F. Max Müller, *Life and Letters of the Right Honourable Friedrich Max Müller*, vol. 1, p. 61.

80. M. C. M. Simpson, *Letters and Recollections of Julius and Mary Mohl*, p. 223.

81. Froude's *Nemesis of Faith* is a novel about a divinity student who gives up his ministry because he cannot reconcile himself to various tenets held by the Church of England, including the Incarnation and Atonement. The book was publicly burned at Exeter College when Sub-Rector William Sewell discovered it in the possession of a student (Basil Willey, *More Nineteenth Century Studies: A Group of Honest Doubters*).

82. Müller, *Life and Letters*, vol. 1, p. 311. Some years later Williams's discussion of Bunsen's biblical researches for *Essays and Reviews*, which refuted traditional interpretations of scripture, resulted in Williams's indictment on charges of heresy (see below).

(God) which is particularized in the various forms of life, the idea that natural laws imply an ordering Mind, the existence of suprasensual knowledge beyond that of the body, that one's will is dependent on one's condition, reincarnation, the cyclic nature of existence, and that evil is a part of the divine plan and remedial in purpose. Many of these ideas are also discussed by Nightingale in *Suggestions for Thought.*

Nightingale and the "Broad Church"

Among Bunsen's English friends and acquaintances were a number of liberal Anglicans including Benjamin Jowett, Thomas Arnold, Arthur Penrhyn Stanley,[83] Rowland Williams, Julius Charles Hare, Connop Thirlwall, and Frederick Denison Maurice. Because their opinions on theological matters were neither those of the "Low Church" (or Evangelical), which emphasized scripture and personal religious experience, nor those of the "High Church," which stressed the Church's authority in matters of doctrine, they were regarded as part of the "Broad Church." This term, according to Jowett, was coined by the poet Arthur Hugh Clough (1819–61; see note 106 below), a classmate of both Jowett and Froude and later Nightingale's secretary.[84] Although many so-called "Broad Churchmen" differed on specific theological issues, the term generally designated a group of liberal Anglicans who were united by their critical approach to both doctrine and scripture and by their belief in the freedom of inquiry. Like Unitarians, the individuals comprising the Broad Church sought to emphasize the ethical component of Christianity rather than its doctrines as represented by the Thirty-Nine Articles and the Book of Common Prayer. They took issue with some church tenets, such as original sin, eternal punishment, and atonement, and questioned whether the Bible was divinely inspired.[85] Broad Churchmen generally held that divine revelation had been imparted to mankind over the course of human history, and was therefore not exclusive to Christianity:

83. Arthur Penrhyn Stanley (1815–81) became Dean of Westminster in 1864 and was criticized for his introduction of Broad Church policies.

84. Charles Richard Sanders, *Coleridge and the Broad Church Movement*, p. 7. Although some, such as Jowett, Maurice, and Thirlwall, objected to being classed under the term "Broad Church," most agreed on freedom of inquiry and the right to express their opinions on matters of theology.

85. Dennis G. Wigmore-Beddoes, *Yesterday's Radicals: A Study of the Affinity Between Unitarianism and Broad Church Anglicanism in the Nineteenth Century.*

... the moment we examine fairly the religions of India and of Arabia, or even those of primaeval Hellas and Latium, we find they appealed to the better side of our nature, and their essential strength lay in the elements of good will which they contained, rather than in any Satanic corruption.[86]

Similarly, Florence Nightingale wrote:

To know God we must study Him in the Pagan and Jewish dispensations as in the Christian . . . this gives unity to the whole—one continuous thread of interest to all these pearls.[87]

Common to Broad Churchmen was their familiarity with German theology, philosophy, and historical scholarship, particularly the works of Schleiermacher and Niebuhr. Having been friends of both, Bunsen played a pivotal role in the Broad Church movement in England. Bunsen himself was the subject of an essay written by Rowland Williams in the highly controversial work of the Broad Churchmen entitled *Essays and Reviews*. The Broad Church movement culminated in the publication of this work, which appeared in print in 1860, the same year as *Suggestions for Thought*. Common to all the discussions in *Essays and Reviews*[88] was the demand on behalf of the clergy for freedom of inquiry in matters of theology and scripture. Noting the ever-widening abyss between official Church positions and those of its more educated members, Benjamin Jowett remarked in his essay "On the Interpretation of Scripture" that "the healthy tone of religion among the poor depends upon freedom of thought and inquiry among the educated."[89] The essayists concluded that theology must be subject to the same rigorous critical analysis as other academic disciplines, and that philosophical, scientific, and historical investigations must be admitted into discussions of theology. To this effect, essayist Frederick Temple remarked: "There are more things in heaven and earth than were dreamt of in patristic theology."[90]

The responses to *Essays and Reviews* were copious and unrelenting: over one hundred responses in print were elicited from members of the Church.[91] With the publication of Darwin's *Origin of Species* just three

86. Rowland Williams, "Bunsen's Biblical Researches," in *Essays and Reviews*, p. 51.

87. Quoted in Cook, *Life of Florence Nightingale*, vol. 1, p. 74.

88. Contributors included C. W. Goodwin, Benjamin Jowett, Mark Pattison, Baden Powell (1796–1860), Frederick Temple (1821–1902, Headmaster of Rugby, later Archbishop of Canterbury), Rowland Williams, and Henry Bristow Wilson.

89. *Essays and Reviews*, p. 373.

90. "The Education of the World," *Essays and Reviews*, p. 44.

91. Josef L. Altholz, "The Mind of Victorian Orthodoxy: Anglican Responses to 'Essays and Reviews,' 1860–1864."

months prior to that of *Essays and Reviews*, the Church obviously sensed that its teachings were under attack and acted accordingly. Essayists H. B. Wilson and Rowland Williams were tried and found guilty of heresy before the ecclesiastical Court of Arches in 1862. (The Church was dealt a serious blow when they were later acquitted by the Judicial Committee of the Privy Council, a state rather than church body.) In 1863 Benjamin Jowett was tried before the vice-chancellor's court at Oxford. Although the charges were eventually droppped, Jowett was denied an increase in his stipend until 1865. In addition, his appointment as Master of Balliol College was blocked until 1870.[92] Ten years after the publication of *Essays and Reviews*, the theological climate was still such that Frederick Temple was forced to withdraw his essay from subsequent editions, following his appointment as Bishop of Exeter.

The Church and its institutions did not take criticisms from this constituency lightly: blatant rejection of Church doctrine by clergy and academics would cost many their reputations and offices. When F. D. Maurice expressed doubts on the Church's doctrine of eternal punishment in his *Theological Essays* (1853), the Council of King's College, London dismissed him, deeming his opinions to be of "dangerous tendency, and likely to unsettle the minds of the theological students."[93] Thomas Arnold and A. P. Stanley were never to receive bishoprics. Max Müller probably lost the election to the chair of Sanskrit at Oxford because of his association with Bunsen and the Broad Churchmen, and thus decided against contributing to *Essays and Reviews*.

Although both *Essays and Reviews* and *Suggestions for Thought* addressed such issues as the critical evaluation of scripture, the implausibility of miracles in a lawful universe, and the doctrine of eternal damnation, only *Essays and Reviews* garnered the wrath of ecclesiastical authorities because the unpublished *Suggestions for Thought* remained discreetly in the hands of a select few. To a great extent the controversy surrounding *Essays and Reviews* was due to the fact that six of the seven essayists were ordained clergymen in the Anglican Church, some of whom had previously aroused suspicion because of their unconventional views. Benjamin Jowett, for example, had been asked by the vice-chancellor of Oxford to renew his pledge to uphold orthodox Church doctrine as expressed in the Thirty-Nine Articles as a result of the views he expressed in his edition of the Epistles of St. Paul (1855).

92. Peter Hinchliff, *Benjamin Jowett and the Christian Religion*, pp. 62ff.

93. Frederick Denison Maurice, *The Word "Eternal," and the Punishment of the Wicked*, p. vii.

Nightingale had much in common with the people who comprised the Broad Church: like them she wanted religion held to the same critical standards as science, philosophy, and history, and like them she had been influenced by German theology. She too challenged belief in the atonement, incarnation, eternal damnation, baptismal regeneration, and miracles. In addition to her friendship with Bunsen, her social and intellectual circle included several prominent Broad Churchmen and liberal Anglicans, including Frederick Temple, F. D. Maurice, A. P. Stanley, and later Benjamin Jowett.

Nightingale had known Temple (also a friend of Jowett, Arthur Hugh Clough, and Stanley), as early as 1852.[94] She probably met Maurice through his sister Mary, who served on the governing committee of the Institution for Sick Gentlewomen in Distressed Circumstances where Nightingale worked as superintendent in 1853.[95] Nightingale was keenly interested in Maurice's quarrel with the Church (see Chapter 4, "On Sin and Evil"), and Maurice himself visited her on at least one occasion in 1855.[96] She became acquainted with Arthur P. Stanley through his sister Mary, whom she had met in Rome, and who was also interested in hospital work and later served in the Crimea.

In addition to her friendships with the above, Nightingale was also familiar with the works of Baden Powell and Mark Pattison, two well-known Broad Churchmen who contributed to *Essays and Reviews* and whom she cites in *Suggestions for Thought*. Yet, despite her associations with these individuals and her familiarity with German theology, the vast literature on the Anglican Church in the nineteenth century nowhere mentions Nightingale in the Broad Church context. The opinions expressed in *Suggestions for Thought* will show, however, that she should be regarded as part of this movement, and that she was commenting on some of the most hotly disputed issues facing the Anglican Church in the nineteenth century. In many instances, her remarks parallel or anticipate those made by prominent theologians like Jowett, Stanley, and Maurice, although it cannot be determined what influence, if any, she had on these individuals.

Nightingale's comments on questions of theology should not be taken lightly. As we have seen, one's religious affiliation and opinions were serious matters in Victorian England. "Dissenters" and Catholics were

94. *Calendar of Letters*, 3.A7,554.
95. *Calendar of Letters*, 3.E4,720.
96. Parthenope Nightingale to Florence, 8 December 1855. Quoted in Cook, *Life of Florence Nightingale*, vol. 1, p. 266.

prevented from holding public office until the repeal of the Test and Corporation acts (1828) and the Catholic Emancipation Act (1829), and Jews were barred from Parliament until 1858. Undergraduates matriculating at Oxford were required to subscribe to the Thirty-Nine Articles of the Church of England, and Cambridge required a declaration of membership in the Church of England as a condition for taking a degree. Connop Thirlwall was promptly dismissed from his tutorship at Cambridge in 1834 for writing a pamphlet in which he advocated the admission of dissenters to the university. The University of London, chartered in 1836, was open to all men "without distinction," but dissenters were finally admitted to Oxford and Cambridge only in 1854 and 1856 respectively,[97] and it was not until the Universities' Test Act of 1871 that the universities of Oxford, Cambridge, and Durham were opened to all men regardless of religion. (Degrees at London were not open to women until 1878, nor at Oxford and Cambridge until 1920 and 1921 respectively.[98])

Theological debates continued to rack the Anglican Church as it struggled to preserve its traditions in the face of scientific and historical investigations and political reforms. By the end of the nineteenth century progressive ideas had gained some ground, and "the opinions of the authors of *Essays and Reviews*, or most of them, became acceptable as well as legal."[99] Because *Suggestions for Thought* remained unpublished, Nightingale's spiritual and philosophical writings, however notable and unique, went virtually unnoticed, unlike her achievements in nursing and public health. In his book on science and religion in the Victorian Age, Basil Willey named "three great explosions . . . which rocked the fabric of Christendom and sent believers scuttling for shelter": Darwin's *Origin of Species*, the Broad Church's *Essays and Reviews*, and John Colenso's 1862 *Pentateuch and Book of Joshua Critically Examined*[100] (see Chapter 1, "On the Concept of God"). If *Suggestions for Thought* had been more widely known, undoubtedly it would have been the fourth.

The Manuscript

Florence Nightingale's spiritual interests and her desire to help the people in the working classes converged in the writing of *Suggestions for Thought*.

97. Owen Chadwick, *The Victorian Church*, vol. 1, p. 480.
98. Joan N. Burstyn, *Victorian Education and the Ideal Womanhood*.
99. Chadwick, *The Victorian Church*, vol. 2, p. 106.
100. Basil Willey, *Darwin and Butler: Two Versions of Evolution*, p. 9.

Nightingale probably made her "curious acquaintance" among the artisans of the north of England[101] while caring for the ill in the villages of Derbyshire, and in London through her friendship with Mrs. Truelove, a publisher and vendor with her husband of radical and "free-thinking" literature. In the late 1840s Nightingale frequented their shop to assess the type of literature that appealed to intelligent working class people. Concluding that the majority were on the road to atheism, she felt challenged to present religion to them in a new way that would appeal not only to the intuition and emotions, but also to the rational mind.

It is generally believed that Nightingale began writing her religious text in 1851–52. This date is supported by letters written to Samuel Gridley Howe[102] and Henry Manning in 1852 in which she makes mention of the operatives of England and the growth of infidelity among artisans.[103] She noted in a letter of 1860 that her "large and very curious acquaintance among the Operatives of the North of England," which prompted the writing of *Suggestions for Thought*, had occurred eight years previous.[104] As we have already seen, the early 1850s seem to have been a particularly stressful time for Nightingale. Family tensions were reaching a crisis level as Florence struggled to answer her calling. She had journeyed to Italy (1847–48) and Egypt (1849–50) in an attempt to defuse the explosive domestic situation and to the hospital at Kaiserswerth (1850 and 1851) to realize her vocation. In 1852 she considered converting to Roman Catholicism. It was in this air of discontent that *Suggestions for Thought* was born.

By the end of 1852 she had a 65-page proof privately printed.[105] It consisted of three chapters, the first entitled "On Law" and the other two serving as clarifications of the first. Much of this material did find its way into the final edition of *Suggestions for Thought*. The proof was put aside when she left England to study nursing in Paris and was not taken up again until 1858, two years after her return from the Crimean War. It was partly

101. Broad Churchman Thomas Arnold was also struck by the physical and spiritual conditions of the working class while traveling through northern England. His observations are expressed in his "Letters on the Social Condition of the Operative Classes," *Miscellaneous Works*, pp. 171–248.

102. Dr. Samuel Gridley Howe (1801–1876), American philanthropist and husband of the reformer Julia Ward Howe, author of the "Battle Hymn of the Republic." The Howes were friends of the Nightingales and visited Embley in June 1844.

103. *Calendar of Letters*, 3.B2,583; 3.B11,610.

104. BM Add. MSS 45768.f112. A reference in *Suggestions for Thought* to Pope Gregory XVI (d. 1846) suggests, however, that Nightingale may have begun work on her manuscript as early as the 1840s.

105. Bishop and Goldie, *A Bio-Bibliography of Florence Nightingale*, p. 119.

because of the interest and help of Arthur Hugh Clough,[106] who was serving as her secretary at that time, that she resumed work on her "Stuff."

The finished work, comprising 829 octavo pages in three volumes, was printed in 1860 by William Spottiswoode, a friend of both Max Müller and Benjamin Jowett, whose company had also printed some of Bunsen's work in England. Although she wrote that she never intended the work to be published during her lifetime (or at least not with her name),[107] she had six copies printed; they were sent to her father, John Stuart Mill, Benjamin Jowett, Sir John McNeill,[108] Monckton Milnes,[109] and her uncle Samuel Smith.

In its original form *Suggestions for Thought* comprised three volumes. The first volume introduces the main ideas; the second volume, subtitled "Practical Deductions," reiterates concepts introduced in the first volume "in the hope of reaching different minds" and includes considerable social criticism; the third volume, the "Summary," simply restates ideas contained in the previous volumes. This format is thus not unlike the proof, in which the second and third chapters expounded upon the first. The complete title of the first volume was *Suggestions for Thought to the Searchers After Truth Among the Artizans of England.* Benjamin Jowett objected to this narrow appeal and urged her to write for people of all classes, because "there is one intellectual world with common ideas."[110] She must have come to the same conclusion, as the second and third volumes were both simply titled *Suggestions for Thought to Searchers after Religious Truth.* She may have also decided to change the title because her social criticism was leveled at the upper as opposed to the working classes, or perhaps she realized that the writing style was not appropriate for artisans. Indeed, Jowett told her more

106. Clough (see above) had been one of Thomas Arnold's most favored and brilliant students when the latter was headmaster at Rugby. In 1852, at the invitation of American transcendentalist Ralph Waldo Emerson, Clough traveled to the United States, where he undertook lecturing and translations of Plutarch. Upon his death in 1861, Nightingale remarked: "He was a man of rare mind and temper. . . . He helped me immensely, though not officially, by his sound judgement, and constant sympathy" (*Calendar of Letters*, 8.B6,716).

107. BM. Add. MSS 45768.f112.

108. Sir John McNeill (1797–1883), a medical officer in the East India Company, met Nightingale in the Crimea, where he had been sent to inquire into the supplies for the British Army. He was an ardent supporter of sanitary reform and later became a trustee of the Nightingale Fund.

109. See note 64 above.

110. Letter from Jowett to FN, 17 November 1861; quoted in Quinn and Prest, *Dear Miss Nightingale*, p. 13. Jowett had received a copy of the manuscript from Arthur Hugh Clough. Jowett's and Nightingale's correspondence about *Suggestions for Thought* developed into an extraordinary friendship that lasted until Jowett's death in 1893.

than once that she should try to present her views in a more readable manner:

> There is always in your writings much that is original & of great value, but it is often not written in a manner suited for the Public & might lead to misconception."[111]

Jowett recommended that she edit the book before publishing it, correcting the tiresome repetitions and digressions. Annotating his copy, J. S. Mill indicated that some parts of the text should be confined to notes as "they interrupt the tenor of the argument & send the reader's mind wandering among the mysteries of Christianity."[112] He encouraged her to go ahead and publish the work, but wrote that "in point of arrangement, indeed, of condensation, and of giving as it were, a keen edge to the argument, it would have much benefitted by the recasting which you have been prevented from giving to it."[113] Recognizing both the defects and the merits of the manuscript, Sir John McNeill wrote to her:

> I doubt whether it is now in such a form as to be extensively studied by the classes for whose use and benefit it is chiefly designed, but I do not doubt that it is a mine which will one day be worked by many hands and that much precious metal will be drawn from it.[114]

Heeding the recommendations of Jowett, Mill, and others who read Nightingale's work, we have condensed and eliminated sentences, paragraphs, pages, and whole sections of the text that were redundant, superfluous or unclear. The remaining material has been reorganized so that discussions of similar subjects, originally scattered throughout the three volumes, are now gathered under new chapter headings. Throughout the editing process, we have *not* altered or paraphrased Nightingale's words: the content, grammar, syntax, and tone remain hers. Indeed it was her combative tone and harsh criticisms of contemporary religion and society that Jowett hoped she would soften:

> Shall I say one odd & perhaps rather impertinent thing? You have a great advantage in writing on these subjects as a woman. Do not throw it away but use the advantage to the utmost. In writing against the world . . . every feeling,

111. Letter from Jowett to FN, 17 November 1861, p. 258.
112. BM Add. MSS. 45840.
113. "Florence Nightingale as a Leader in the Religious and Civic Thought of Her Time," p. 79.
114. BM Add. MSS. 45768.f120.

every sympathy, should be made an ally so that with the clearest statement of the meaning there is the least friction & drawback possible.[115]

Jowett valued her work, however, and wrote that he would be very sorry if the greater part of this book did not in some form see the light: "I have been greatly struck by reading it, and I am sure it would similarly affect others. Many sparks will blaze up in people's minds from it."[116]

Suggestions for Thought should not be seen as a complete or finished work. Rather than presenting a unified, cohesive philosophy, it comprises Nightingale's thoughts, observations, and ruminations on a variety of religious, philosophical, and social concerns. Indeed, the title *Suggestions for Thought* indicates the conversational tone of the text. Derived in part from personal correspondence to friends and relatives, it is at times sarcastic, flippant, and prone to exaggeration and generalization. She corresponded at length on religious subjects with Julius Mohl, as mentioned previously, and also with her father's sister, "Aunt Mai."[117] As Cook notes, "Aunt Mai" had considerable talent for metaphysical thought and was of help when Nightingale started writing *Suggestions for Thought*.[118] Nightingale herself admitted to Aunt Mai's influence: ". . . without you dearest Aunt Mai, I am certain I should never have thought of these things—or any of the things which are now most interesting to me."[119] Passages from letters to family and friends were actually integrated verbatim into the text, contributing to its unwieldiness.

The original work included copious margin notes that did little to enhance the organization of the material and have thus been omitted in this edition. The lengthy digests that preceded each volume were merely compendia of the margin notes and thus have also been omitted. The author's punctuation and use of capitalization (which are inconsistent) and use of italics have been retained here.

In our commentary we have chosen not to write a critique of Nightingale's ideas because this would require a separate, lengthy philosophical discussion. We have endeavored only to clarify her ideas and in some cases to provide a historical or biographical context for her remarks. Likewise, we have not attempted to present a complete comparison between her views and those of other philosophers. Our commentary, clarifying re-

115. Jowett to FN, 17 November 1861; Quinn and Prest, eds., *Dear Miss Nightingale*, p. 13.
116. Quoted in Cook, *Life of Florence Nightingale*, vol. 1, pp. 472–473.
117. Mary Shore (1788–1889), W.E.N.'s sister, married to Samuel Smith.
118. Cook, *Life of Florence Nightingale*, vol. 1, pp. 120–121.
119. BM Add. MSS. 45793.f75.

marks, and any text other than that written by Nightingale are clearly distinguished by typeface. Our notes are numbered consecutively through each chapter; Nightingale's own notes are indicated with asterisks. In editing *Suggestions for Thought* we have endeavored to do that for which Nightingale never had the "time or strength or inclination"—that is, to present her work in such a way as to make it accessible to the educated public. We have tried to be true to Nightingale's ideas and to the spirit of the work, and we hope, as did Jowett, that "many sparks will blaze up in people's minds from it."

Michael D. Calabria
Janet A. Macrae

Suggestions
for Thought
by Florence
Nightingale

DEDICATION.
TO THE ARTIZANS OF ENGLAND.

Fellow-Searchers,

I come to you not to declare the truth; I come to ask you (if subjects of moral truth have an interest with you) to join in seeking it with those capabilities which God has given to us. I offer the result of my own endeavors, and what I am able to gather from the endeavors of others.

The object of our desire is to be Truth. All should have their faculties exercised and educated, for the purpose of forming a judgment of what is God's truth.

It is thought desirable for all to learn what is necessary to gain a livelihood. Arithmetic and other matters of instruction are taught for this purpose. But education is not pursued altogether with a right spirit and purpose. Man's education should be given for the purpose of re-generation; of putting him in possession of the capability of exercising his powers, so that those powers may reveal to him what, among the labors of mankind after truth, is really truth; may enable him to judge of the nature of God, the nature and destination of man, and how practically to pursue that destination.

But how forlorn, many say, thus to be left without an authority on the awful subject of religion!

We are not left without "authority." The Spirit of Truth will be our authority, if we will faithfully seek Him. Can there really have been an "authority," when such different Gods have been believed in; such different modes of serving God pursued? Truth is, indeed, One; but the only way to "unity of faith," is a true cultivation of the nature, and a true life in which to exercise it. If this can be discovered, unity of faith will exist.

Moses and Paul came forth from their desert, saying, "this and this is miraculously revealed truth, which the world is to believe." Should it not rather be said, "this is truth, viz., that man is to discover from the means within and without his nature, all the truth to find which that nature is competent"?

We offer you what we believe to be truth. We offer our reasons to your reason, our feelings to your feeling. Judge ye if it is truth.

Do we speak of what is important? Then consider it. Is it important? If not, hear us no further in this matter.

I. On the Concept of God

What do we mean by "God?" All we can say is, that we recognize a power superior to our own; that we recognize this power as exercised by a wise and good will.

I

Nightingale begins by commenting on the state of religion and, more specifically, the Anglican Church in the mid-nineteenth century. She describes an age of spiritual uncertainty when some, fearing that scientific and historical investigations of the Scriptures would destroy their religion, sought refuge in the authority of the Church. Her comments to this effect are well-grounded in historical reality, and allude to the so-called "Oxford Movement." Championed by John Henry Newman and Edward Bouverie Pusey, the Oxford Movement sought to emphasize the Catholic essence of the Anglican Church. Embracing the doctrine of apostolic succession, Newman held the authority of the Church even above that of the Scriptures:

Surely the sacred volume was never intended and is not adapted to teach us our creed. . . . From the very first, the rule has been, as a matter of fact, for the Church to teach the truth, and then appeal to Scripture in vindication of its own teaching.[1]

Promulgating their views in a series entitled *Tracts for the Times*, Newman, Pusey, and their supporters became known as "Tractarians." Censured by the vice-chancellor, heads of houses, and proctors of Oxford, and denounced by many Anglican bishops on account of the views he expressed in Tract XC ("Remarks on Certain Passages in the Thirty-Nine Articles," 1841), Newman grew increasingly dissatisfied

1. Quoted by David Newsome in *The Victorian Crisis of Faith*, p. 81.

with the Church of England. His confidence in the efficacy of the Church was finally shattered in 1841 when a joint Anglo-Prussian bishopric was established in Jerusalem through the efforts of Baron von Bunsen.[2] This action effectively linked the Church of England with German Protestants, whereas Newman was seeking common ground between Anglicans and Roman Catholics.[3] Newman's conversion to Roman Catholicism in 1845 prompted the departure of many Anglicans to the Church of Rome, including the wife of Nightingale's friend Sidney Herbert.[4] (Herbert himself had been a "Puseyite"—a follower of Pusey. In *Suggestions for Thought* Nightingale sardonically refers to Puseyism as the "calm before death."[5])

From all indications, the Church of England was in turmoil. Parliament had effectively curbed Anglican political prestige by extending the civil liberties of Roman Catholics and "dissenters" (non-Anglican Protestants), Newman was leading Anglicans to Roman Catholicism, and German rationalism was taking root in England where it threatened Church doctrine. That the Church perceived these "new-fangled doctrines" (as Nightingale alluded to them) as a threat is evident from the title of Pusey's first book: *An Historical Enquiry into the Probable Causes of the Rationalist Character lately predominant in the Theology of Germany* (1827). A further indication of the crisis was the 1851 census of religion, to which Nightingale refers in her text. The census indicated that of the nearly 18 million people comprising the populations of England and Wales, some 5¼ million who were physically able to attend a house of worship did not. In addition, half the individuals attending services were dissenters.[6] Church attendance was lowest in the large manufacturing districts, less than 25 percent of the area population.[7] Thus it is to this group in particular, the "artizans," that Nightingale dedicated *Suggestions for Thought*. Painfully aware of the crisis in the spiritual life of the culture around her, in which people either

2. See discussion in the Introduction above.

3. According to the terms of the agreement, the bishop of Jerusalem would be nominated alternately by the British and Prussian governments. He would be consecrated according to the Anglican rite, and would ordain Lutherans who accepted both the Anglican Thirty-Nine Articles and the Lutheran Augsburg Confession (Marvin O'Connell, *The Oxford Conspirators: A History of the Oxford Movement, 1833–1845*, p. 351). For Newman's objections, see his *Apologia Pro Vita Sua: being a history of his religious views*, pp. 133ff.

4. Quinn and Prest, *Dear Miss Nightingale*, pp. 50–51.

5. *Suggestions for Thought*, vol. 1, p. 180.

6. Chadwick, *The Victorian Church*, vol. 1, pp. 363–69.

7. K. S. Inglis, "Patterns of Religious Worship in 1851."

indiscriminately embraced orthodoxy or adopted rationalism and renounced religion entirely, Nightingale sought to reconcile these two extremes.

*   *   *

Look at the state of theology now. Multitudes of conscientious and feeling persons, terrified at the work in which the mind of the age is engaged, in sifting opinions long taken for granted as true, fearing that, if those opinions were lost, all religion would be lost, are ceasing to reason, sheltering themselves under authority.

Many are speculating, some as an amusement, some with real earnestness, on the very defects of theology as now taught.* Such a word [speculation] is entirely unsuited to the subject, which should engage our deepest thoughts, and should lie at the foundation of the whole of our practical life. On such "speculation" we have no desire to enter. Our object is real practical progress for mankind through true religious belief. We hear of the "rise and fall" of empires. Now one country, now another, is in the ascendant. We hardly know why or wherefore. Real continuous progress for mankind at large will only be through men uniting to learn from God's laws what man ought to be, how men ought to live—through their uniting to bring about that so men shall be, so men shall live.

But people will discuss the merest trifles interminably, and leave such questions unsettled, as why man is what he is, none caring to know. Could mankind but reach mankind's sense upon the matter, and compare each other's opinions, some progress might be made. But everybody is afraid of everybody else on this subject; men of being thought to sap the "foundations of religion;" women of being thought pedantic and presumptuous;

---

*Scarcely a day passes but books, by the orthodox and the unorthodox, by men and by women, are advertised, with titles as follow (I take these at random):—"Passing Thoughts on Religion," "Musings on Manifestations of God to the Soul of Man." As for the "Impressions," the "Aspirations," their name is legion. Now, can we call this anything byt *impertinence* to God? What should we say if we saw advertised, "Passing thoughts" on hydrostatics, "Musings" on clinical surgery, "Impressions" on life assurances? Everybody would laugh, and nobody would read the book. Is religion, confessedly the most important of all subjects, to be the only one on which anybody's *passing* thoughts are good enough? Is the nature of God the only science not worth study? I am not aware that any book called "*Fancies* on Religion" has yet appeared, but the title would be by no means a misnomer, for much that is written consists of nothing but fancies. A life of the Virgin Mary, which I have read, in eight volumes, called "*La Cité Mystique de Dieu,*" by a Spanish nun, who believed it to be the work of inspirritation in her, is not mre the work of fancy than are some of these Protestant effusions.

religious professions of saying anything but upon authority. Thus nothing is said and little thought upon the matter.

"What *is* the religion that people have now?" If they do wrong, they say, Let us pray—pray for pardon and peace. If they have "trials," as they call them, they say, Let us bear them patiently: in another world it will all come right. If they are well-meaning and conscientious, and they make mistakes, or fail, or are hindered by external circumstances, they say, God takes the will for the deed: in heaven we shall see our hopes fulfilled;—not, there will be no heaven for me, nor for any one else, unless we make it— with wisdom carrying out our thoughts into realities. Good thoughts don't make a heaven, any more than they make a garden. But we say, God is to do it for us: not we. We?—what are we to do?—we are to pray, and to mean well, to take care that our hearts be right. "God will reward a sincere wish to do right." God will do no such thing: it is not His plan. He does not treat men like children: mankind is to create mankind. We are to learn, first, what is heaven, and secondly, how to make it. We are to ascertain what *is* right, and then how to perform it.

Duty is so difficult now; formerly it was quite certain what there was to be done. People were to go to church and teach their children the catechism and the creed, and give away flannel petticoats and broth, which was called "doing good;" there was no doubt about it. But now it is truly said of many a woman, "she has been trying all her life to do a little good, and has done a great deal of harm." People know that giving away is not doing good, and they don't yet know what to do in its place; even such a school as King's Somborne is not doing unmixed good. No more do people know what to teach their children; even the atheists among the operatives cannot bear teaching them that there is *no* God, and yet they do not know *what* God to teach them. A religious woman used to attend "Divine Service" on Sundays and say her prayers, that was her religion. Her goodness was to be careful of the poor, and to do little kind things by everybody, and further, to make society for her children; about all these things there was no doubt; but now?...

Good people often say that they are afraid of all these new-fangled doctrines destroying spiritual feeling, cutting off communication with God. But what have they now? what communication have men, have gentlemen, with God? They go to church because their wives make them, and criticize the sermon a great deal, and they have prayers with the servants in the morning, because their wives wish it; but no one ever thinks of *this* religion as a religion for men, but as one for women and children.

Has the House of Commons much communication with God? It reads its prayers every day, it is true.

It is said that we could have no comfort in our religion if we did not think our prayers were heard and answered.

Surely *that* is the most *uncomfortable* part of it. You say your prayers and you don't know whether God has heard you or not, whether He will answer you or not, nor *why* He has heard you, nor how to bring Him to answer you. Some few feel, from the sensation of comfort and satisfaction in themselves, that He has answered them; other few are miserable because no such feeling in themselves gives them a conviction that He has heard them. The greater part go their way, having "done their duty" in "saying their prayers," and never look for any result at all.

This morning I read to my dear grandmother the Psalms for the day, as usual; I sang "unto the Lord a new song," I sang "praises unto his name;" "For why?" as the Psalmist very properly asks; why, indeed? Because the Lord had killed all the young Egyptians, both human beings and animals; because he had favoured the Israelites and proscribed every one else. So do we think now, viz., that He "hath set apart" the English for Himself, and favoured them to the detriment of every other nation. And, really, that such things should be "sung and said" by educated men in every church in England "throughout the year!" Two hundred years hence what will be thought of us? that we ought to have been in a lunatic asylum; but people in lunatic asylums are more sensible. Is it as extraordinary that a man should think himself a teapot as that we should think God like this?

In this age, atheism and indifference are man and wife. In former times, atheism used to be the father of despair. But now people live without God in the world, and don't so much as know that He is not there: they are not aware of his absence. Formerly, the terror and the anguish of the sceptic testified to what he had lost, and were the truest witnesses to God and to his own *religiousness*. Now, the indifferentist is called the religious man, and the religious man is the heretic.

Indifferentism, satisfied with conventional life, busy in gratifying man's external pleasures, prevails largely. Among the earnest spirits, the resource is, either a return to Roman Catholicism, or "let us work at our lives, and leave alone this subject of religion, which only makes men quarrel."

How do you know a religious man now? By his going to church. And going to church is considered as a duty, that is, as something *due*—to whom?—to God: something you have done for Him; He is flattered by your going to church. But it is not always done as a compliment to Him; sometimes it is done as a compliment to our fellow creatures. Mrs. A. is deaf, and cannot hear the service; but she always goes to church for the sake of "example." A great many ladies never miss going where they are known, for this purpose; but if they are where they are not known, they do not go. What a poor compliment it is to God to go, not because you have something you want to say to Him, but "because Mrs. A. goes." In a country church, if there is a wedding of any consequence, the church is always sure to be full the first Sunday the bride appears, in order to see her. "To see the bride," is a very innocent amusement; but is religion come to that pass in this country that people go to a place, where they say they expect to meet God, to "see the bride?"

In more civilized society, a woman scarcely ever leaves a breakfast table to put on her bonnet for church, without hearing a joke among the men and the inquiry, "Shall *you* go this morning?" "No, I don't like the Litany. Shall you?" "Yes, I shall; I don't like shocking our hostess." And when you meet at luncheon, "Have you fulfilled your ecclesiastical duties? Oh! shocking; don't you consider it a duty? I did not know you were so bad." Or "I counted forty-six people asleep this morning."

And when one thinks that there are fifteen thousand sermons to be preached this morning, and more than fifteen thousand breakfast tables where similar jokes are making,—and this is called a Church, and this religion!

The feeling of the Church of England is very intelligible. Many know that they are in a state of "twilight faith." But what can they do? If they stop out of it, they step into a state of darkness. They have not admitted the principle, "Search," and it is like stepping out of a rickety house into the blank cold darkness of unbelief.

Is it not possible that this sense of uncertainty it is which has led so many lately into the Roman Catholic Church, and some the most learned, the most earnest? Scepticism, not belief, has brought them there. They required their sense of a truth to be stronger and more complete than it was. The more they urged themselves to believe, the less real was their feeling of belief, till, at last, they took refuge in the belief of others to supply that which they had not in themselves.

In this age, however, by far the greater proportion of mankind, have gone the other way; in England, most of the educated among the operatives, especially in the northern manufacturing towns, have turned their faces to atheism or at least to theism,[8]—not three in a hundred go to *any* place of worship; the moral and intellectual among them being, almost without an exception, "infidels." What the most conscientious among our working men seem to be doing now, is renouncing religious error, not announcing religious truth; they seem not to be seeking after light, but giving up darkness.

These poor fellows, thinking so hard and so conscientiously, leave out the best element in the food which they so earnestly seek; the most divine element, that which makes confusion into order, that which makes the lowest into the highest; for the highest discoverable principle in existence, perhaps, is the feeling residing in the perfect One, which wills happiness; the thought of the perfect One, that happiness is, by its essence, worked out for the happy by exercise of their own natures and of other natures like theirs. *Time* is all that intervenes between man as he is, and man made one with God.

II

Nightingale continues her critique of contemporary religion and prevailing concepts of God. Here she briefly takes issue with the practice of prayer, the Scriptures, and doctrines such as the Incarnation, Trinity, and Atonement, all of which are treated in greater depth in subsequent discussions. Although she finds fault with virtually every religious denomination and sect, she does occasionally make mention of their good qualities, and does so in the following discussion for Roman Catholicism. In spite of Nightingale's unorthodox views, this comes as no surprise as she herself considered converting to Catholicism in 1852.[9] Deeply attracted to the Roman Catholic religious orders devoted to serving the sick and poor, she was for the moment able to ignore the confines of Catholic doctrine. As will be seen however, her praises for Catholicism are quickly followed by strong criticisms.

*   *   *

8. Theism is the belief in an omniscient, omnipotent, and personal God deserving of worship and obedience. Nightingale objected to the idea of a personal God who intervened in human affairs at will (cf. Chapter 2, "On Universal Law"), and found worship in the sense of praising God inappropriate. See her comments on "Worship" in Chapter 6, "On the Spiritual Life."

9. See discussion in the Introduction.

But most of all do we not want our God? Is he not our first want? The Roman Catholic's God is not ours. To live very closely with those who are all worshipping very fervently one God, while we are thinking about another, and that other not at all like theirs, is very painful. To have sympathy with our God, to be able to esteem Him is surely the first thing. To live with those who are worshipping not at all fervently another God, still less like ours, because He is so far off and we are so very indifferent about him, is more painful still. The God of any church now existing is a different God from ours.

It is so easy now, men can have no religion and not know it themselves, because it is all laid down for them what they are to think and what they are to say; their services are not with them a matter of feeling. The Dean of ———— and the Bishop of ————, while labouring so intensely in the cause of humanity; have they any religion? And yet they don't know themselves that they have none, when saying their services. They never think of asking, because they have no doubt they have.

People have no God now. A few speculate as an amusement to the intellect, but most have a diluted religion of the kind of St. Teresa's.[10] They use the prayers she did, but without expecting the answer she did. They pray for rain, but they look at the barometer and ask which way the wind is. What can you expect of a religion which uses the forms without awaiting the result? They pray indeed, but they don't know whether they shall have it or not. If they have, they are surprised; if they have it not, they say it was not wise to give it them. But our God always does what is wise, whether we suggest it to Him or no. St. Teresa was so much better than her God.

The Protestants, it is said, do not feel so much for their purer God as the Catholics do for their unjust one.

But we can hardly call the Protestant God a God at all. What does He stimulate us to do? What does He require of us but to go to church once a week? We cannot say, "Why are the Protestants not better than the Catholics, their God being so much less absurd?" We can only say, the Protestants have hardly any God at all. They were so occupied with the absurdities of the Roman Catholic God that, as often happens, they did not perceive that they had left themselves no God at all. For the last 300 years, the work of religion has been a work of destruction.

10. Nightingale was somewhat critical of the Spanish mystic, St. Teresa of Avila, because she saw Teresa's God as capricious rather than lawful (see Chapter 2, "On Universal Law"). Nevertheless, she was deeply interested in Teresa's writings and planned on incorporating some of them in her *Notes from Devotional Authors* (see Introduction, p. xiii).

And when will it come to be a work of edification?

Even now we hear "the voice of one crying in the crowd, 'Prepare ye the way of the Lord.'"[11] We do not wonder at the rejection of Monotheism on account of its dullness. The Jewish religion and the Unitarian are the dullest of all. They are pure Monotheism. The Catholics, with their angels, and devils, and Saints, and Virgin, and the Holy Ghost, and the Son, do make religion more exciting. But God in his solitary existence, enjoying while we are suffering, is the most cheerless religion—would be revolting, if we really believed what we think we believe. No wonder we turn from him with indifference and then complain of our hard hearts. But all that the Catholics have we shall have as soon as we have made them. Every man is not intended to be superior in every thing. But, let him organize a right life, and men superior to himself in different things (or "angels") will spring up. And mankind, not only Christ, will be the Son. A great sacrifice has been made for us; God is suffering for us—not enjoying Himself by Himself. Our religion will have everything.

The Incarnation—the Trinity—the Atonement seem to be abortions of a comprehension of God's plan. The Incarnation? We do not see that God is incarnate in *every* man. We think He was only incarnate in one. We make the Trinity God, Christ and the Holy Ghost—instead of making it God and man, and such manifestation of God as man is able to comprehend.

The Atonement? Man had a dim perception of God passing through sin and suffering for man and in man, and also of sacrifice and compensation—though it seems a curious sort of compensation that His Son should suffer and die because we have offended Him—the whole scheme of grace and redemption appears to be an elaboration of error founded upon some truth. And yet this is believed, and the simple scheme of God's providence men are so scandalized at; it is indeed necessary to have a church to keep up all this.

"How glad we should be, if God *did* speak to us, as St. Teresa thought He did," is often said.

But there is hardly anything which it has ever been *supposed* that God did say, than which we could not have said something better ourselves. What St. Teresa says,—what Moses says,—the ten commandments—are they not full of mistakes? "I am He that brought thee out of the land of Egypt." He was taking care of the Egyptians as much as of the Hebrews. "I

---

11. Cf. Matthew 3:3, ". . . the voice of one crying in the *wilderness* . . ."

the Lord am a jealous God." The iniquity of the fathers *is* indeed visited upon the children, but not because God is "jealous." The fifth Command-ment[12] contains three mistakes, first, we *can* only honour that which is honourable; secondly, filial piety has nothing to do with living to old age; thirdly, the Lord did not give them that land (in the sense in which Moses said it)—they took it. As to "Thou shalt not kill," "Thou shalt not steal," we did not require a voice from God to tell us that it was better not to kill and steal. Christ does *not* say that God spoke. It shows his great wisdom. But, in the few times when God is said to have spoken in the New Testament, it does not appear that He said anything very inspiring. He said, "This is my beloved Son, in whom I am well pleased, hear ye Him." When he speaks to Paul, and says, "I am Jesus whom thou persecutest," we feel sure that that is *not* what He would have said.

It is true, there is much in the Christian religion which has nothing to do with Christ.

The atonement, the incarnation, these *He* never preached—nor the ecclesiastical pomp, nor the fabric of the hierarchy.

Nothing, in the vagueness of people, strikes one so much as their raving against the Catholic superstitions, and not seeing that, if the words of Christ were exactly followed out, the Catholic Orders will result—the parting with all they have—the leaving father and mother—all excepting their mortifications,—those He never preached.

The orthodox took hold of a great truth, when they got hold of the incarnation—but they confined it to one—they did not extend it to all. They dwell so much on the passion of Christ, which He suffered for us for a few hours, and they think nothing of the passion of God for eternity—which He suffers for our sakes since the world began. Books upon books have been written upon the day's suffering, till the most fanciful schemes have been built upon it, as might be expected, in order to supply materials for thought. If they would think upon the plan of God, the sufferings of God from eternity, what truths might not be discovered! what mines are there not to be worked! The gospel of a perfect God. What a gospel might be preached!

The "evangelicals" so often complain of their hard hearts, (Wesley's[13] whole tone is of nothing else) they say they cannot love God. Is it any

---

12. "Honor your father and your mother, that your days may be long in the land which the Lord your God gives you" (Exodus 20:12).

13. John Wesley (1703–1791), founder of Methodism.

wonder? How can they love the being whom they imagine? They work themselves up by excitement into a kind of spasm of interest about Him; but they must find their hearts hard, in a religion so essentially cold.

It seems to be inconsistent with love and wisdom to have the work and the suffering to any but itself; therefore God works for us in us. The true feeling of *God in us*, which led to the belief of one incarnation, ought to be extended to the incarnation *in all of us*.

The Roman Catholic idea is not nearly so fine as God's thought. But it is the *next* fine idea to it. If God had not done what He has done, He would have done what the Roman Catholics say He has, that is, if He had not made truth discoverable by the exercise of man's faculties, He would have *told* it to man in one continuous line of communication and revelation, as the Roman Catholic church says He has to her. It is curious, however, that the whole cumbrous fabric of contradictions,—contradictions to love and wisdom—should be thought right and orthodox, when compared with the simplicity of God's scheme, at which people are "shocked."

Mankind have thought a great deal about doing the will of God, but have not thought *what* God is and *what* His will will be—what he will like—when they try to do it.

And now people think less of what will be the will of God than of what will gain the sympathy of men. Now, too, in times when what God likes, and what men will sympathize with are so very different—when, in truth, what God and man will sympathize with, is hardly ever the same thing—this is dangerous indeed.

III

Ideas make progress. And the meanings attached to words which express ideas cannot, therefore, remain the same.

A house may mean a house in all ages, though even in the case of words which express things, the house which we build now signifies a very different thing from the house built from the painted Briton. How much greater must be the difference in the sense of a word used to express a religious or a political idea! Either we must have new words or new meanings.

The word "God" has been used to express such various conceptions that there is a degree of vagueness in the proposition, which, however, we admit to be undeniable, since all those conceptions include the idea of super human power.

It would be the greatest gain religion has ever made, if, for a time, the word *God*, which suggests such various and irreverent associations (irreverent, that is, to a spirit seeking right,) could be dropped,—and the conception substituted of a perfect being, the Spirit of Right.

*   *   *

From Nightingale's point of view, science is not opposed to religion but is actually necessary for the attainment of religious truth. She explains below that the conception of a perfect being, the Spirit of Right, is evolutionary. With the advancement of culture (in science as well as the arts), humanity awakens to the idea of a perfect God, who is the essence of justice, wisdom, and goodness, as well as of power.

John Stuart Mill, one of the first to read Nightingale's manuscript, did not share her belief in a righteous God. In a letter to her (September 23, 1860), he wrote:

> There are many signs in the structure of the universe of an intelligent power wishing well to men and other sentient creatures. I could, however, show, not so many perhaps, but quite as decided indications of an intelligent power or powers with the contrary propensity. . . . It may be that the world is a battlefield between a good and a bad power or powers, and that mankind may be capable, by sufficiently strenuous cooperation with the good power, of deciding or at least accelerating its final victory.[14]

As will be seen in subsequent chapters, the concept of a benevolent God is the basic premise of Nightingale's spiritual philosophy. "The whole doctrine of a future state depends on it," she wrote, "and all our capability of perfection."

*   *   *

Here we come to consider the meaning or rather the meanings with which the word "God" is used. It has been used to signify the most different ideas in different ages and nations. Can you attach any similarity of idea to the God whom his people whipped to make him do what they liked and to

14. Quoted in "Florence Nightingale as a Leader in the Religious and Civic Thought of Her Time," p. 80.

the God who sat enthroned in the mystic phrase of Zoroaster? Nothing is more common than to say, there never has been a race nor an age which did not believe in a God. *A* god certainly. But *what* God? What does the word mean? A cat?—a lamb?—a spirit?—a statue? These words are as synonymous as the different Gods in which different races and different ages of the same race have believed. When you ask, Why do you believe in God? I must ask, Which of the ideas of God do you mean? whether the God of the Old Testament, who commanded the extirpation of the Canaanites? or the God of the New Testament, who commanded submission to the yoke in many things in which, as we worship Him now, we believe that He commands the struggle for freedom?

The God "of Abraham, of Isaac, and of Jacob," was certainly *not* the God "of the whole earth." It is true that the Hebrews *served* but Him alone; they *believed*, however, in the existence of many Gods. Their own God they reverenced, and despised the other Gods. But it was not till long afterwards that they rose with increasing knowledge to the belief that there was but one supreme. Yet He cannot be perfect if there be more than one. Is it, perhaps, that a knowledge of natural philosophy, such as cannot be attained by an infant nation, is necessary for the conception of one supreme being? The more we learn the more cause we find to think that the whole system of the universe is one scheme. Astronomy leaves no room, so to speak, for more than one throne. The same legislation prevails everywhere. All becomes one whole, with one ruler.

Man advances to a consciousness and conviction that there does exist a perfect being (whom we may call God), exactly in proportion as his nature is well constituted, well educated, well exercised. Human nature, when thus *well-born* and *well-bred*, will *admit* of his sense of this truth, and of others inferred from it, being as strong and complete as the sense of truth with which he asserts that the tree before his eyes is a tree, and not a house.

But we must be careful to know that the God whom we believe in *is* a perfect being. Men often think that they believe in a perfect God when, in fact, they do not,—when they are really wholly incapable of even conceiving of a perfect being. For instance, in the earlier nations, where revenge was considered a virtue in man, it would naturally be thought so in God. Many imperfections, as we now think them, were once deemed virtues, and consequently attributed to a God who was *called* perfect.

Authority does not teach belief in a perfect God. It is evident that very few have believed that their God was perfect. Some nations have not professed to do so; others have attributed to him qualities essentially imperfect, while giving him the title of perfect. For instance, the Greeks did not suppose their Zeus, Athene, &c. perfect. They attributed to them merely human qualities with superhuman power. Athene was the goddess of wisdom, not the wise goddess. Themis was the goddess of justice, not the just goddess. So our Perfect Being is goodness, is wisdom, is power.

In these earlier nations, *power* seems to have been the principal characteristic of a God. He or she was merely an engine to account for creation. Take all the thousand different meanings, which have been attached to the word "God" by different nations and individuals in different ages, and some kind and degree of power above human seems to be all that is common to them. In these days we profess that we believe our God to be perfect, but we attribute to him all kinds of qualities that are not—love of His own glory, anger, indecision, change of mind—and we try to believe, if we think at all, that a God with these qualities is perfect.

Man's conscious weakness, the terrible sufferings he has endured which he has been powerless to prevent, the intensity of his desire for what he cannot obtain, his imperfect conception of moral right, have confused might and right. Power to do what he cannot do has been his God.

The earliest and still recurring question of man concerning the Superhuman Power which he dimly recognizes seems mainly to have been how to obtain that this Power shall assist his desires, relieve his sufferings. He does not conceive of this Power as acting on a principle, or according to a rule. He attempts to propitiate Him by offerings, by sacrifice, by glorification, by prayer; or, believing in the moral nature of God, he supposes human suffering the result of God's displeasure for man's sinfulness. He believes, for instance, that cholera may be removed by man's repentance for sin, averted by his refraining from it. He has not recognized that to the virtuous or the vicious cholera is incident in certain states of body, under certain circumstances.

✳   ✳   ✳

The idea of God "acting on a principle" is Nightingale's way of reconciling science and religion. The perfect God expresses Himself through universal laws as opposed to divine caprice. In a lawful universe, actions generate consequences, and thus propitiating God is impossible. The righteous God, however, did not leave human beings without help in their suffering because He gave them the power of understanding. Human beings are to discover the laws of God and to alleviate suffering by properly applying them. The perfection of mankind can thus only occur by means of a synthesis of the spirit and the intellect.

While writing *Suggestions for Thought*, Nightingale consulted the works of the philosophers Sir William Hamilton[15] and Henry Longueville Mansel[16] in order to see what she did *not* believe.[17] Whereas Hamilton and Mansel had concluded that man was incapable of perceiving the Divine, Nightingale held that God's laws revealed His nature (see Chapter 2, "On Universal Law"). Nightingale briefly addressed Hamilton's views in an appendix to the first volume of *Suggestions for Thought*.

*   *   *

Religion is a feeling towards a *good* being. We have believed that *power* gave rights, and we have worshipped a being with power, but not with goodness. Should we call fear of a devil a religion? Can we call Calvin's a religion? A God who, for no other reason than His own "good pleasure," predooms some beings to happiness for eternity, and some to misery for eternity; or a God who destroys some of His children for the benefit of others.

It is the common mistake that might makes right. The clay must not say to the potter, "why didst thou make me so?" But the conscious intelligence *may* and ought to question its Maker's ways, and say if they are according to right. Because He is more powerful than we are, is that a reason why He should do according to His fancy? It is an old confusion between might and right. At first some power greater than human was all that was recognized, then almighty power; and it was thought that that power gave the powerful the right to do anything he pleased, and that the clay, the vessel, must not question it. "Shall the clay say to him that fashioneth it, what makest thou?" It was not perceived that He has the

15. Sir William Hamilton (1788–1856), Scottish philosopher, professor of logic and metaphysics at the University of Edinburgh.

16. Henry Longueville Mansel (1820–1871), English theologian and philosopher, systematized William Hamilton's work. In *The Limits of Religious Thought Examined* (1858) he denied the possibility of knowledge of the absolute and was thus accused of agnosticism.

17. BM Add. MSS. 45790.f180.; Letter to W.E.N., 16 July 1860, Claydon Collection (*Calendar of Letters*, 7.B3,354).

power, and could not have other than the will, to do everything which is *according to* wisdom and goodness, He being goodness and wisdom himself.

We are to understand the nature of God, and we can make no progress without such understanding. The whole doctrine of a future state depends upon it, and all our capability of perfection.

If you would, therefore, let me leave the question, why do you believe in God?—as not knowing which of these ideas of God you mean—I would say instead, I believe that there is a Perfect Being, of whose thought the universe in eternity is the incarnation.

It is evident that every nation, every age, *could* not believe in a Perfect Being—that it required cultivation, development to conceive the idea of perfection, and that the higher all the faculties of an individual, as also of a nation, have been, the higher has been his conception of God, the nearer perfection.

It is true, some of those called the most highly cultivated of the human race, Descartes,[18] Laplace,[19] Hume,[20] have not been able to conceive of a God at all.

But, have they been the most highly cultivated? Only intellectually so. And it seems evident that the *intellectual* idea of Him is *not* the highest. That is merely reducing Him to a master engineer, a mechanician-in-chief. Is not goodness for this purpose higher than intellect? Has not the innocent child probably an idea of God nearer the truth than that of Voltaire or Gibbon? "Unless ye become as little children, ye shall not enter into the kingdom of Heaven." We believe the carpenter's son, who humanly did not know that the earth moved round the sun, to have had a truer conception of deity than the philosopher, who had fathomed the laws of creation.

18. René Descartes (1596–1650), French mathematician and philosopher. Descartes actually did argue for the existence of God as a first cause. He defined God as infinite and perfect, liable to no defect or error. In annotating his copy of *Suggestions for Thought*, J. S. Mill pointed out Nightingale's error: "There must, I think be some mistake here about Descartes. He not only believed but thought he had proved the existence of a God *a priori*" (BM Add. MSS 45840.f11). She acknowledged his remarks and thought that her error could be deleted from a revised edition.

19. Pierre Simon de Laplace (1749–1827), French astronomer and mathematician, famous for his celestial mechanics and also his theory of probablility, which he applied to social problems. Demonstrating the internal stability of the solar system, he found no need for divine intervention or maintenance.

20. David Hume (1711–1776), Scottish philosopher and historian. Known for his scepticism, Hume refuted various arguments for the existence of God. Although he attributed an intelligent design to the universe, he did not accept the ideas of a benevolent God, the immortality of the soul, or the truth of the biblical tradition.

But he would have had a still truer, if he had known all that Laplace could have told him.

The more highly man's moral, intellectual, and spiritual faculties are cultivated, the more nearly will he approach a true conception of God. But of reason, feeling, and conscience, feeling, truly cultivated, is that which gives us the truest conception of God; though, of course, a harmonious development of *all* these faculties would give us a truer still.

Thus the goodness of God is a Higher attribute than His wisdom or power.

The question, Why we believe that there exists at all an Eternal Spirit of perfect goodness, wisdom, and power, I can only answer, By experience, and experience only. What mankind can learn of the past, the present, and the future is in harmony with the existence of such a spirit; without it, is unaccounted for. In earlier ages it was thought that what we see about us could not be accounted for, except by supposing imperfect qualities in the Eternal Spirit. But if,—as we make progress, we find a great many marks that He is perfect,—if by degrees we should find that that very evil, which had made us *doubt* His perfection, is one of the truest proofs of it, shall we not come at last to think that He has done in the universe what we should have done, had we been perfect?

Thus increased knowledge, knowledge of the laws of God, is essential to our forming this idea of His perfection. Although a man in a dark room may often form a truer idea of Him than a philosopher observing the rotation of the sun, still, besides a man's *feeling* of what is *right*, his power of comprehending providence depends on his knowledge of the past, the present, and the future.

If it be said that this is reducing the wise and good God to the measure of my own understanding and heart, I answer, Not to mine, but to the accumulated and accumulating experience of all mankind.

IV

Nightingale explores the meaning of religion, contrasting her view with that of Auguste Comte, the French positivist philosopher whose ideas she gave much consideration (see Chapter 2, "On Universal Law"). Although she shared some of his views with respect to empirical science, because her cosmology was implicitly theocentric she was disturbed that so many artizans were embracing his atheistic philosophy.

Nightingale maintained that a true understanding of religion required the operation and integration of *all* human faculties—physical, intellectual, affectional, and spiritual—which would replace Church doctrine and Scripture as the means of discerning truth.

Although she spoke of the "deep truths" contained in the Bible, scattered throughout *Suggestions for Thought* are pointed remarks, such as those already encountered in Section II, which clearly indicate that she refuted the Scriptures as divine revelations. In a letter to her father, she wrote: ". . . there are cruel mistakes in the Sermon on the Mount, tho' it is quite possible that Matthew put them there."[21] Because portions of the Scriptures contradict what we know of universal law, they cannot, in her opinion, be true revelations:

Our disbelief in these [the Bible, Qur'an, and others] as direct revelations, *i.e.*, as being other than man's noble attempts (up to the present time) in the course of his development, to understand God, (in which attempts he has formed "God in his own image,") is founded on the contradiction in these to universal law.

This once admitted, what have been supposed to be revelations, cease to appear so, because, on this admission, they fundamentally contradict both what "is" and what "ought to be."[22]

In concluding that science, history, and the collective experience of mankind are the means of discovering religious truth, Nightingale was in agreement with the Broad Churchmen, particularly Benjamin Jowett, who held that

any true doctrine of inspiration must conform to all well-ascertained facts of history or of science. The same fact cannot be true in religion when seen by the light of faith, and untrue in science when looked at through the medium of evidence or experiment.[23]

Flagrant criticism of the Bible was a serious matter, especially when it came from the Church's own constituency. For denying the divine inspiration of the Bible in *Essays and Reviews*, Rowland Williams and H. B. Wilson were charged with heresy.[24] Their case was soon followed by that of John William Colenso, Bishop of Natal, South Africa.[25] Deposed in 1863 on account of his *Pentateuch & the Book of Joshua*

21. BM Add. MSS. 45790.f312; *Calendar of Letters*, 10.B12,466.
22. *Suggestions for Thought*, vol. 1, p. 216.
23. *Essays and Reviews*, p. 348.
24. See discussion in the Introduction.
25. See discussion in the Introduction.

Critically Examined (1862–1879), Colenso sought to prove "the un-historical character . . . of the five books usually attributed to Moses." Although the Judicial Committee of the Privy Council ruled in his favor, Colenso was nevertheless excommunicated by the bishops of South Africa in 1866.

＊   ＊   ＊

What is the meaning of the word "religion?" Is it not the tie, the *binding*[26], or connexion between the Perfect and the imperfect, the eternal and the temporal, the infinite and the finite, the universal and the individual?

In Comte's works, religion is nothing but the state of perfect harmony proper to human existence, collective as well as individual, when all its parts are fittingly co-ordinated.

This is not religion, but that which would be the effect of religion. Religion is the connexion of the heart of the imperfect with the Perfect. The seat of religion is in the heart. It will call forth all the energies of the intellect to demonstrate the Perfect, all the activities of all the nature to accord with the Perfect in life.

The essence of religion is love of a living good and true and right,— veneration, admiration, trust, sympathy in a good and true and right above human.

The primary fact in religion seems to be the existence of an omnipotent spirit of love and wisdom—the *primary* fact, because it is the explanation of every other.

This gives us four words to explain, each of which is open to great misconception, and has been greatly misconceived; viz., omnipotent, spirit, love, wisdom.

By *omnipotence* we understand a power which effects whatever would not contradict its own nature and will.

By *spirit* we understand a living thought, feeling, and purpose, residing in a conscious being.

By *love* we understand the feeling which seeks for its satisfaction the greatest degree and the best kind of well-being in other than itself.

By *wisdom* we understand the thought by which this satisfaction is obtained.

---

26. Nightingale is referring to the possible derivation of the word "religion" from the Latin *religare*, "to bind."

But, first, is religion a subject to be logically treated, or is there any truth in the feeling of deprecating, as irreverent, the sifting of what is true, as to religious belief, by the aid of the science of logic?

If religion is to depend upon evidence, not upon intuition or consciousness, a more comprehensive evidence is required than is necessary for any other subject. More faculties must be exercised for this purpose than are required in seeking after truth on any other subject. If a man is seeking truth in physical astronomy, the perceptive faculties alone will enable him to draw his inferences. But he will not know thus all that is to be known about astronomy, or the most important part of what is to be known about astronomy; for that most important part is its relation with religion.

But with what faculties are we to inquire? The Germans on the continent, and Mr. Newman[27] at home, say that there is a special faculty which they call the *soul*, or "intuition" (*anschauung*), which apprehends God, which knows Him, as the senses know the external world. There is a school (Unitarianism as it was) which says that this faculty is *intellect*, and that man apprehends religious truth by a process similar to that pursued in any other scientific investigation. Mr. Martineau[28] has looked to the moral nature of man, and shown that man cannot appeal to his *conscience* without coming to religion.

Why should Mr. Martineau, or Mr. Newman, or the intellectual school, expect to find religion revealed by *one* faculty, independent of others? If we wish to estimate a man rightly, to hold right intercourse with him, all our faculties are wanted. We shall not rightly estimate mankind, or live well among mankind, unless every faculty we have is in exercise. Should it not be so as to religion? A man will be really religious in feeling and act, will apprehend religion rightly, in proportion as *all* his capabilities are rightly exercised, and in proportion as the society in which he lives is organized so as to afford full and free exercise for his nature.

There have been three parties—those who have said that there was a revelation through the book; those who have said that there was a revela-

---

27. Francis William Newman (1805–1897), the liberal brother of Oxford Movement leader John Henry Newman, and author of *The Soul* (1849) and many other religious works. He was unable to take his MA at Oxford as he did not subscribe to the Thirty-Nine Articles, and subsequently became a Unitarian (*Dictionary of National Biography*, supplement 3).

28. James Martineau (1805–1900), philosopher and Unitarian minister, brother of Harriet Martineau. He favored the use of intuition and human conscience to discern religious truths, rather than adhering to Church doctrine or Scripture. In *The Rationale of Religious Enquiry* (1836), he wrote: "Reason is the ultimate appeal, the supreme tribunal, to the test of which even Scripture must be brought." It is undoubtedly this work to which Nightingale is responding.

tion through the Church, or through the book and the Church; and those who have said that there was no revelation at all. Now we say that there is a revelation to everyone, through the exercise of his own nature—that God is always revealing Himself.

Let us suppose that we give up the usual means of receiving truth from church or book, and that we seek it from God through our own faculties, including the spiritual, the affectional, the intellectual, and the physical; and including what these can receive from God by means of the same faculties in mankind as well as in our individual selves. It seems important that the thinkers of the present day (men disgusted with church and book as authority) should be fully aware of this; understanding, however, that from book and church we may learn, inasmuch as therein is also to be found exercise of human faculty.

We believe that *all* the faculties of all mankind should be exercised to receive the revelation of God to man. The Roman Catholic, the Anglican, &c., &c., &c., exercise a very limited number of faculties in what they receive as revelation.

If the eye is diseased, we see falsely; if the reason, feeling, &c., are so, we judge and feel untruly. In both cases we must take care to keep our sources of information in a healthy state. "If thine eye be single thy whole body shall be full of light." "If any man shall do His will, he shall know of the doctrine whether it be of God" or not. If you will carry your belief into your practice you will soon find out whether it is true.

We agree with the Roman Catholic, that is dreadful to be without authority. But we *have* authority. Is not God Himself authority? We are but the vessels. He fills them; and we must keep the vessels unsoiled and pure.

It is said that those who do not admit "authority" do not know *when* it is God that speaks, and when it is the excitement of a cup of coffee—that they cannot tell whether their vessel be pure. Swedenborg's was pure, and St. Francis of Assisi's was pure, yet they came to different conclusions. We may naturally be mistaken in what God says to us, because we have to construct for ourselves and each other the vessel into which the Holy Ghost enters, and often inevitably it becomes occupied with other ghosts. It is truly remarkable, indeed, how some have believed that Christ said to them what they said to themselves, and this with the printed book before them. Little, indeed, does that book probably represent Christ—as little as other books of men's sayings and doings represent *them*. Still, it assures us that he did not think what he has since been said to have thought.

Will it be said that it is presumption and conceit for a few individuals to think that they can discover the true nature of religion, and how it ought to be manifested in life? There is no fear of such presumption, for according to the nature of things, no such conceptions would come into the mind of individuals till *mankind* had been long, long and laboriously at work. Comte profoundly teaches that the errors in man's view of religion are essential paths to truth—they have been no wild vagaries, independent of law. Our heads and our hearts should estimate them with the respect and affection due to them. While we sift truth from falsehood in books held sacred, which have come down to us, let us estimate the value of the truth— the truthfulness, *in its position* as to time and place, of the falsehood. How short-sighted, feeble, and vain is he who fancies *himself* individually to have discovered anything! How disgusting is the narrow selfish folly of A, who is contending in angry pages that he, and not B, made a certain discovery! Be assured it was neither A nor B—it was mankind, it was God in man. The perceptions or ideas in A's mind could never have arisen had not a thinking and laborious race preceded him. When, therefore, you strive in the glorious work of endeavouring to read the revelation of the Great Spirit in time and space, fear not to be presumptuous in using the capabilities which that Spirit has bestowed for this very purpose; fear not that you are arrogating to yourself a power above other men. All science, all history and experience of human nature, which the ages of man have laid before you, are your means for discovery.

"The Church of England is a good human help," it is said. What does she offer as help? She has certain prayers taken from the Roman Catholic, which, if you find that they suit your feeling too, you may go and hear every Sunday; twice, if you like; in some places every day; and you may hear the Bible read, which some say you can do just as well at home; and you may hear a sermon preached by the best educated in the land, educated in classical literature, Aristophanes and Cicero, and such theological learning as we can give. Few *men* attend to the sermon, but they may criticise it. Farther, you may be married, that is, have a form of words pronounced over you, which makes your marriage the law of the land; and you may be buried, or the feelings of your friends gratified by having certain words read over you; and when you are ill you may send for the clergyman to read a service by you; and you may receive the sacrament once a month; and your children may be baptized. This is the help the Church offers, which we may take if we like it.

The Church of England has for men bishoprics, archbishoprics, and a little work (good men make a great deal for themselves). She has for women—what? Most have no taste for theological discoveries. They would give her their heads, their hearts, their hands. She will not have them. She does not know what to do with them. "You may go to the Sunday school, if you like it," she says. But she gives no training even for that. She gives neither work to do for her, nor education to do it, if she had it to give. Many women would willingly give her their life's work. Luther gave us "faith," justification by faith, as he calls it; and the Church of Rome gives us "works." But the Church of England gives us neither faith nor works. She tells us neither what to believe nor what to do.

But the Church of England may make discoveries, may make progress, it is said. The Roman Catholic Church cannot.

The Church of England is no training for a discoverer in religious truth; we might as well say that a mathematician is prepared to enter upon farming, as that a man trained in Latin and Greek, and theological learning, is prepared to find out truth in religion. When we walk through the new House of Commons, those rooms do not look like the rooms of an assemblage of men straining to find out truth for a great country, political truth, or the good of a nation. Nor does the Church look like an assemblage of men fitted to find out religious truth.

If it is asked, "Are we capable of finding out truth?" it may be answered, that what we *might* be is indicated by moments. We are surprised to find the depths of feeling we are capable of. If life were organized so as to produce constantly what we are now conscious of at moments, "eye hath not seen" that which man might do. And, instead of talking about man being "desperately wicked," we should say, as we sometimes do say of great heroes, we did not know of what man was capable. Instead of that hideous hopeless repetition every day for years of "there is no health in us,"[29] we should be living with a purpose, a purpose of moral improvement, which would be constantly realized till we were "perfect, even as God is perfect." What a difference there is between those thus living with a purpose and those who live with no purpose at all! These take up a book, but not with any particular object to further. They have no purpose but amusement.

Our religion is too exclamatory to be a religion. All our prayers begin with "O Lord," as if we were trying to excite in ourselves a feeling which we have not.

29. From the Book of Common Prayer.

V

There is great interest in tracing the derivation of words. It is a means of tracing man's thought. It is interesting to think concerning each word that there was a time when it had never been used, to ask the question, of what thought, emotions, or sensation was it the consequence, when it first passed the lips of man.

The word *truth* appears to have been derived from *troweth*—that which a man believes was *trowth* or truth. And here we see into a common error of mankind. Often man does not look for the absolute *what is*, but satisfies himself with that which he "troweth." Nay, many go so far as to assert that there is a different truth for different natures. If we mean by truth *that which is*, we mean a definite mode of existence not subject to be changed by the view which different men take of it.

But, among the different views which men take of religion, is one, then, only true?

All are imperfect; none without some true belief, if, by true belief, we mean belief of that which is. The conception, the comprehension, of the Infinite and Perfect which the finite and imperfect struggles for must always be, like himself, finite and imperfect, but, like himself, it may be ever advancing and improving.

It has been said that man makes his God. He does so in an obnoxious sense, if he supposes that he conceives and comprehends the whole truth concerning God in his creed, be it what it may. He who fashions a figure of wood, and then bows down to it, is called an idolater. We are shocked that, by his limited faculties, he has limited the conception of the superhuman power. When man limits his conception of the superhuman power by any form of words, he makes the same sort of mistake as the man who fashions an idol with his own hand. Let us ever remember that our conception, our comprehension, our feeling of God must be ever imperfect, yet should be ever advancing.

We must not *make* God: we must *find* Him and feel Him more and more. "He that loveth not knoweth not God." How imperfect our love, how imperfect our wisdom, to fulfil the purpose even of such love as we feel! In proportion as we partake the attributes of God, shall we know Him better. Love and knowledge must unite. He who feels and comprehends, by his feeling, God's love, will know God better and better as he penetrates into His wisdom, as revealed and revealing itself in the everlasting tale of the universe. The nature and history of the material, the intellectual, the spiritual will all be to him, as he learns them, revelations of God. Love, without knowledge, will form a poor conception of God; knowledge without love will form none at all.

Were we in geography or astronomy to take one book as our final rule, our ultimate appeal, the same thing would happen inevitably as has happened in religion. Some things in it we should absolutely ignore, as when we ignore that Solomon said, "Man is like the beasts that perish;" and of other things we should say, "he did not mean that—he meant something else;" as when Christ says, "Hate your father and mother, sell all, and follow me." No one would cry out so much as the bibliolaters—"what a shame!" if we were to *do* it; but they say "he did not *mean* it." Could we go on with such a system in geography or astronomy?

And yet there are things which nobody does really believe. Suppose I were to say, "consider the laurel of the garden, how it grows! It toils not, neither does it spin. Do you do like the laurel, and you will have food and clothing too." People answer, Christ did not mean that, he meant something else. Yet such is the vagueness of men, that this is preached one day in the seven, and the other six days the board of guardians preaches something quite different.

The people look and see, and they see that practically the guardians are right, and that Christ was wrong, and some are frightened and say, "I have lost my Christ;" and others are hardened and say, "I don't want your Christ." These are two alternatives, equally unsatisfactory; but if we put in juxtaposition with this "the kingdom of Heaven is within," or some other of the truly divine things which Christ has said, and feel that after all there was no one like him, none who knew so much truth as he did, none who lived as he lived,—than we are neither hardened nor frightened; we do not lose the truth, and we have not to lie to ourselves about the untruth; we can truly say, never man spake as he spake.

Many who do not believe Christ miraculously inspired do not become hardened about him; they love him more that ever they did; they admire his life and character more than those do who think him God.

But many men who never read the Bible, because their common sense resists such things as "Take nothing for your journey, neither scrip, nor staff, neither bread, nor money, nor even two coats;"[30] and "Shake off the dust against any who do not receive you;" things which belong to the times

---

30. This must have particularly bothered Nightingale, who saved countless lives in the Crimea by her foresight in obtaining provisions.

of the Essene communities, but not to these, and which do not even sound perfectly just and good, as belonging to *those* times,—men who cannot bear to read these things, will yet be shocked at not thinking Christ divine. Divine? We too think him divine as all men are divine, but not the *only* divine One. As he said himself, "those are Gods or the sons of God to whom the word of God comes."

The Unitarians say that no man is divine, none an incarnation of God; the Trinitarians that there was one. What do we mean by a man being divine, or an incarnation of God? Are not all men "incarnations" of God, in proportion as they receive truth as truth is to God, as they think His thought, partake His consciousness, are one with Him? Do not all men partake this blessed *one*-ness in proportion as in them are kept the conditions on which, in accordance with God's will, it depends? So strong is our conviction of this that in so far as to recognize divinity in one man is better than in none, Trinitarianism is truer doctrine that Unitarianism.

*   *   *

Nightingale was clearly a Platonist. Unlike modern existentialists, who maintain that truth is only what we as human beings create,[31] she speaks of an objective Truth or Meaning which transcends and is independent of the human mind.

Does not what we recognize of existence call upon us to believe that there is a thought, a sentiment, a purpose which comprehends all existence? Such a thought and purpose certainly exists in no man, nor in all mem put together. For all mankind long thought themselves living on a flat stationary surface. Whose thought and purpose, then, was this star among stars revolving round the sun? Can this question be avoided?[32]

Nightingale firmly believed in the evolution of human understanding and in the mind's capacity to arrive at ultimate Truth. When she speaks of an eventual "unity of faith," therefore, she is not speaking of unity within any existing church. She is referring to an evolution of human consciousneses through which all human beings will realize "the beauty of God's plan." The search for religious truth is impeded, Night-

31. See, for instance, H. J. Blackham, *Six Existentialist Thinkers.*
32. *Suggestions for Thought.* vol. 1, pp. 62–63.

ingale forcefully reiterates, by the acceptance of one book or set of teachings as the final authority.

*   *   *

As much as the Roman Catholics can believe that there will be unity and infallibility, so do we. How can the preachers of toleration of the present day say, "take the religion which suits you best," any more than "it *may* suit your mind better to believe that the sun moves round the earth, if so, take the belief which you find best for you?" There may be a mind which, from want of imagination, want of cultivation, cannot be make to apprehend that the earth is not an immoveable body, but one flying through space; and it is true, therefore, to say "there are minds which must believe that the earth is stationary *till* they are more cultivated." But unity in religion there must be one day, as surely as there is unity in astronomy. There is objective truth and untruth in religion, as in astronomy, and the well-constituted mind, by the exercise of its own powers, must and will come to this unity of truth.

It is a mistake to refer us to "private judgment"—those words are dangerous, because they seem to imply that one person may judge one way, and another another, according to their "private" views of things, according as it "suits their own minds," as the phrase is, whereas it is the truth, as it were, which *judges* for us. The principle of "private judgment" ought to mean (if it means anything) that we are to search earnestly with all our mights for the truth, and that *that* is to judge, not that *we* are to judge. The principle cannot be too strongly laid down that there cannot be two truths, any more than two Gods. There can be but one truth; it cannot vary to suit the minds of each. There is but one truth, and we have to find it. The Roman Catholics say, truly, there is but one truth. But some say that we are to find it in the Bible—some that we are to find it in the Bible and Church together. Comparing the churches, some say that we are to find it in the Roman Catholic church, others that we are to find it in the church of England, and some that we are to find it in the Roman Catholic church *or* in the church of England—they are not quite sure which. But we don't want to ask the church. We want to ask God. But God tells different people different things. So it was in astronomy. God has told Sir John Herschel[33] a

33. John Frederick William Herschel (1792–1871), English astronomer.

great many things which He did not tell Galileo, which it was not in Galileo's possibility to receive. Do we complain of this? We do not say that each is to take the system of astronomy which best suits his own mind. Are we not to strive to find out the truth in religion as we have been striving to find it out in astronomy? There is but one truth. Most dangerous is it to allow the belief that there may be two—that is as our "private judgment" judges best. God judges for us, and His truth it is which we have to find out. "Private judgment" is not the question. It is God's "judgment."

There is a truth, and we must find it out. "It is the truth for *you*,"—we don't say this in medical science—we don't say "only believe,—believe sincerely, and it does not signify what you believe—be but conscientious in your belief, that will do." Religion is the only thing which is of so little importance that we can say this. In medical science, we say "it is a matter of the utmost importance to health that you should discover the truth—search for it, then, with all your might; if you don't find it, there may be fatal consequences." But in theological science, and theological science only, we do *not* say "you must bend your whole faculties, to discover and earnestly search out the truth." No, "tolerance" says, "if it be only your conscientious opinion, and if it suit the nature of your own mind, that will do."

Suppose that, in nautical matters, we were to say "I think *so*. You think otherwise. It would be very illiberal of me not to think that you may be right and I be right too. It is better that men should be of different opinions—let each man have his own. Let each take the opinion which suits his own mind and tolerate the other's." Were this said in nautical matters, or were naval men to refer to a chart made in 1300, what would be the consequence? Yet thus it is in religious matters.

"But what test have we, if each man is to depend upon his own faculties?" it is said.

In sanitary science there is a test,—to make the body healthy. But this test does not exist for theological physicians, viz.:—to make the soul healthy. On the contrary. *They* are to say that the soul never can be healthy. It is as if the sanitarian were to say, "You were born in such a state of disease that I can do nothing for you in this world. There is no hope of your ever being well. You will never get better here. Do not, therefore, expect it or strive for it. But I have to announce to you that, by some method which you cannot understand, by the death of a God a long time ago, you will be quite well in a state which comes after the time when you will be dead in this. Only believe this and you will be quite well *then*;—*here* you never can be."

There is one truth, which is God's truth, and we have to find it out and to educate mankind to be capable of receiving it. But "tolerance" says "any religion will do which you yourself think a good thing." Is it for me with my foolish thought to say what is a good religion? It is God's thought which I am to seek for. "But that is the truth for you and this is the truth for me," it is said. "If he only follows his private judgment, it is the truth for him." It is not for him with his "private judgment" to make a truth,—he has to find out what is God's truth. There is but one truth, which all have to find out,—there are not as many truths as there are private judgments and individual minds.

This, it is said, is to go back to the Roman Catholic Church, to "turn back again to the only foundations of certainty, and lay once more" *in her* "the basis of your faith."

Rather it is to *go on* "to the foundation of certainty, and to lay" *at last* "the basis of faith" which must be our object. It did seem no wonder, when men asked whether poor little babes were damned or not, and the church of England said "it was an open question," "it did not signify, you might believe one way or another, as you chose,"—it did seem no wonder that she thus sent so many earnest men, who thought that it did signify, into the Roman Catholic Church.[34]

The Roman Catholics say that the Church of England "prevaricated in her answer." She did not "prevaricate." She said, "she did not know,—it did not signify!" The Roman Catholics say, "ask Gregory[35] what he would have said." But we don't want to ask Gregory; we want to ask God.

Each (by exerting his own faculties) will learn of God who is infallible, the truth. The truth is discoverable, if we will bring our faculties to it as to any other truth. Is it not as infallibly true that a man must not have three or four wives, or that I am not to go into Mrs. M.'s room and take a 5l. note, if I can find one, as that the earth moves round the sun? Does not all educated England believe the one as "infallibly" as the other? Polygamy and theft are wrong as "infallibly" as it is untrue that the earth is stationary. These are discoveries as to the nature of man. These lead directly to discoveries as to the nature of God, which discoveries, when man applies his faculties to make such, instead of pinning them to a book, will be as remarkable as have

---

34. A reference to the Gorham case—see Chapter 4, "On Sin and Evil."
35. Pope Gregory XVI. The fact that Nightingale uses Gregory (Pope, 1831–1846) to make her point, rather than referring to Pius IX (1846–78), who was Pope at the time *Suggestions for Thought* was published, suggests that she began writing the book as early as 1846.

been his discoveries in every other line. So, with the exercise of man's faculties, there will be "unity."

The Roman Catholics say "there must be unity," and they are right, for the want of unity results from some minds not having yet received the truth, not from there being *no* absolute truth. But they say "there must be a church to maintain this unity and to interpret that book." The other way is to say "the more sects the better. Difference in religious opinions is good. Let *me* believe what I like and do *you* believe what *you* like." This is called *liberality* or toleration. Religion is treated quite differently from anything else. We do not appoint a church or assembly in nautical matters, which is to be infallible. But men search and discover. The principle of searching is still unacknowledged in religious things. And as to the other way, it is simply saying that there is *no* "truth."

But, if mankind can find out God by the exercise of their own faculties, how does it happen that we have not long since found him out, that we have not long since a Church dedicated to that search?

Hitherto all the efforts which have been made in religion, since Christ's time, have been either to cut off error, or to believe what you *say* you believe. The Catholics say, "Christ says, be poor like me, leave your family for my sake, *we are going to do it*." And the religious orders are the consequence. The Evangelical party says, "You tell us that Christ died on the cross for us; this really makes a great impression upon us; we cannot go and laugh and dance as if he were not dead." These are the efforts which have been made to act out what *was believed*. Luther and the Reformers were the men who cut off some monstrous errors. *Protestants* they rightly call themselves; for *to protest* was all their business; and there is nothing very high or noble in protesting. To search for truth has yet to be brought forward as an object.

2. On Universal Law

A law is nothing else than a thought of God.

I

The belief of universal and invariable law has necessarily gained ground gradually, because its foundation is observation and experience. To those who in past ages had not the possibility of recognizing law, it was natural to see superhuman power chiefly in the more interesting and startling events of life, and to seek help through prayer or other means, which human experience represented as likely to please or propitiate. Men *could* not then believe what now stands on evidence. They naturally imagined a revelation which satisfied their (then) moral and physical wants.

But more light has been gained, more truth on morals, on physics; and now if we would look, we might find a revelation founded on evidence to all, not on hearsay to a few.

People who inquire on religious matters generally take separate subjects, or whatever may have happened to attract their attention.—"What is the evidence for the existence of a God?"

We have endeavoured to show how vague is this question, since no one word has been used to express such different conceptions as have been included in the word "God."

"Is there a future state?" means often (perhaps generally) is the future state to be, which is alluded to rather than described in the Bible? Are we all to be called to account for our actions, and rewarded or condemned accordingly, to live above the clouds "in the bosom of Christ," "to be called to glory," or to suffer "everlasting damnation?"

The intellect of the day rebels against such belief, but constructs no other.

Or "have there been miracles?" or "how shall this or that passage in the "sacred writings' be understood?" Or questions arise in the various existing churches or religious associations as to particular doctrines or modes of government.

All these questions, pertinent in their day, and to be respected while they were suitable to that phase of human nature, to *that* state of human knowledge, are left behind, if God's universal, invariable law is recognized. And the questions which God's laws reveal to us, as those which we *ought* to ask, which include all others, become those with which we set out.

II

At the time Nightingale was writing *Suggestions for Thought*, the positivist philosophy of August Comte was arousing interest among the intellectuals as well as the artisans of England.[1] Harriet Martineau[2] had made Comte's work easily accessible by publishing a condensed English translation of his *Cours de Philosophie Positive*.[3] George Lewes, the companion of author George Eliot, wrote a popular summary of positivism entitled *Comte's Philosophy of the Sciences*, which also appeared in 1853. Eliot, an acquaintance of Nightingale's who had also become dissatisfied with the present state of religion, held Comte's work in high esteem.[4]

Believing that humanity's search for truth is a developmental process, Comte identified three sequential stages: the theological, the metaphysical, and the positive. In the theological stage, all natural events were attributed to actions of supernatural beings or "gods." In the metaphysical stage, the personal gods were replaced by impersonal yet absolute forces such as natural law, inalienable rights, and so forth. Comte felt that the fatal mistake in both these stages was the attempt to explain natural events in terms of ultimate supernatural causes. He insisted that

1. See Charles Cashdollar, *The Transformation of Theology, 1830–1890: Positivism and Protestant Thought in Britain and America*; also the discussion of Comte in the Introduction to this volume.

2. Harriet Martineau (1802–1876), a well-known author and journalist, contributed to the *Daily News* and the *Edinburgh Review*, wrote books on economics for the layperson, and was an anti-slavery advocate. She corresponded with Nightingale for many years. Although the two women had some differences of opinion on the issues of religion and feminism, Martineau supported Nightingale's plans for public health reform. She used material from Nightingale's *Notes on Matters Affecting the Health, Efficiency, and Hospital Administration of the British Army* for a series of *Daily News* articles successfully reprinted in book form under the title *England and Her Soldiers* (1859).

3. *The Positive Philosophy of Auguste Comte.*

4. Eliot, *The Life of George Eliot*, pp. 411, 721.

the human mind had limitations; it could never know ultimate causes or anything beyond phenomena. In the third, or positive, stage this mistake would be corrected because the search for truth would focus solely on that which is knowable: the observation and analysis of empirical data. In Comte's view, the various fields of physical science had developed through the three historical stages, and the study of social phenomena was about to enter the positive stage. Indeed, Comte is considered to be the founder of modern sociology because he insisted that the scientific method be applied to the study of human behavior.

Nightingale agreed with Comte that human behavior is subject to universal laws, as is everything else in the universe. She profoundly disagreed with him, however, with respect to the origin of these laws. Deeply influenced by Plato and the mystics, Nightingale held that the laws of science (the organizing principles of the universe) emanate from a higher intelligence, the mind of God. "Now, if we could get rid of the word 'law,' we would," she wrote, "and substitute for it 'a thought of God.' For that is all that it means." In this she echoes the remarks of the Danish physicist Hans Christian Oersted (1777–1851) who wrote: "The laws of Nature are the thoughts of Nature; and these are the thoughts of God."[5]

In the philosophy of positivism,[6] reality is defined as only that which is revealed through the senses or measured by physical instruments, the extensions of the senses. This perspective thus excludes a metaphysical or spiritual dimension from which the universal laws emanate. Without the concept of God, Nightingale felt that Comte's philosophy was incomplete and not ultimately satisfying:

A profound mind and a most feeling heart is making converts to a doctrine in no way calculated to satisfy the heart, which, however, needs only to cry aloud for its satisfaction, in order to find that which really exists and, at the same time, to keep all that the profound thought of Comte reveals.

All that needs to be changed to satisfy our consciousness of truth is (but oh! what a change!) the change of a lifeless law for a living spirit of right, and

---

5. From his *The Soul in Nature* (1852), quoted in Peter Addinall's *Philosophy and Biblical Interpretation: A Nineteenth-Century Conflict*, p. 165. That Nightingale was familiar with Oersted's writings is evident from passing references to him in *Suggestions for Thought* not included in this edition.

6. Nightingale's own definition of positivism is as follows: "Positivism is limiting knowledge to phenomena, to 'that which appears,' and to the 'relations of that which appears,' with the admission that we can know nothing of 'that which is.' 'Man's life, in short, is a life,' says Positivism, 'that has to do only with appearances and their relations; it is not his part to inquire concerning existence" (*Suggestions for Thought*, vol. 1, p. 183).

truth, and love. Comte would not deny that the law has *signs* of right and goodness, is (in many respects at all events) what, if a right and good spirit did exist, with power to will such law, that spirit would will.

Let us search then; let us unite to search in a truth- seeking spirit, in a brave spirit, which fears not truth, all of us, whose hearts yearn for a righteous, wise love, to which to attribute the law, which is more and more discerned to govern all existence, to make it what it is. Of this law Comte has been the special declarer. But there he stops.[7]

Comte himself came to the conclusion that human society could not be improved through the work of science alone; something was needed that would appeal to the emotions and bring about personal and social harmony. For this reason he developed a Religion of Humanity, in which the most noble human qualities were the object of worship and an altruistic life the aspiration. For Nightingale, however, the most noble human qualities are but a pale reflection of the character of the Perfect God.

Some biographers have emphasized the similarities between Nightingale's and Comte's views and tried to link Nightingale with the positivists. Nancy Boyd writes that "her empiricism, her love of science, her faith in logic, and her rejection of a supernatural basis for religion all put her in the positivist tradition."[8] Nightingale and Comte clearly held certain views in common, but her basic assumption of a transcendent God, as well as some of her other beliefs such as life after death, the inner divinity of mankind, and the capability of the human mind to apprehend Truth or "that which is," are not at all compatible with positivism. As she herself states in *Suggestions for Thought*: "We repeat very distinctly that we are no disciples of Comte or of Buckle.[9] We yet believe them to be powerful minds, who have obtained an insight into certain important truths, perceived certain errors in the ordinary beliefs of mankind."[10]

*   *   *

There is no cause but God; all the rest is the effect of His laws or thoughts. A certain circumstance brought into contact with a certain na-

7. *Suggestions for Thought*, vol. 1, pp. 180–181.
8. Boyd, *Three Victorian Women Who Changed Their World*, p. 203.
9. Henry Thomas Buckle (1821–1862), English historian and author of *The History of Civilisation in England* (1857–1861). Buckle held that the actions of men, and therefore of societies, are governed by fixed laws, and sought to demonstrate this with the use of statistics.
10. *Suggestions for Thought*, vol. 1, p. 267.

ture, must always have a certain, the same, and a definite effect. It will not have sometimes one effect and sometimes another. Nature and circumstances remaining the same, to say that any other effect will occur is contrary to experience.

The word "law" when it is used to express some regulation of man, includes the idea of will or intention that, *when this is, that shall be.*

By a law of God, we mean that it is a volition of God—that there is, and shall be, constant relation of succession or co-existence with regard to certain modes of being; such as that, coexistent with certain other modes of existence, it shall always be that particles press equally in all directions— thus constituting one mode of being which we denominate a fluid. Our experience is, that such laws are invariable, never broken. "Thou shalt do no murder" is sometimes called a law of God written in the heart of man, or pronounced by God through Moses. But this cannot be said to be "laid down"—to be a volition of God. It is broken many times in every year in the nineteenth century in England and Wales. To call it a volition of God would be to say that God's will is *not* always done.

A law may be kept in various modes or manners. The law of gravitation is kept whether a man falls down a precipice or stands upon the earth. But one mode of keeping God's law is salutary, another pernicious to man's temporary well-being. (We say *temporary*, for the whole of the laws of God is such that temporary evil only is possible. The *whole* of the laws of God is such that they are self-rectifying, with regard to their effect upon man's well-being.)

Now, if we could get rid of the word "law," we would, and substitute for it "a thought of God." For this is all that it means.

How did all existence come to be what it is?

Comte answers, by law.

And come not law by God?

Comte says, there is no other God than law; or, if there is, we can comprehend no other.

This appears to us unintelligible. As little should we have understood if some one, showing us a manifestation of a law of Solon, had said, "In this manifestation of law, you behold Solon; or, if you do not agree to this, at any rate his law only, not himself can you recognize." If Solon had been existing, though not manifested to our senses, we could have revered, loved, his nature, if in his law appeared the manifestation of goodness and wisdom.

Neither do we know what those mean who say that nature *is* God, more than we should if they said, St. Peter's was Michael Angelo. In St.

Peter's we see a manifestation of Michael Angelo. The first stroke which he made in his design had reference to every other; each stroke had reference to each past and future one; or, if not, there was deficiency. It stands as his spirit or nature in manifestation, by means of material nature, to other spirits. So the nature or spirit of God is ever manifesting itself, in the change of the present from the past. The spirit which is ever at work, manifesting itself in accordance with perfect wisdom, goodness, righteousness, order, beauty,—ever comprehending an eternal past and future in the will of the present,—exists in perfect satisfaction, in constant activity. His will is law. His law manifests itself in the existence of the universe as it is, as it has been, as it will be. Both pantheism[11] and "positivism" have a truth, but they leave us still without the all-comprehending thought, sentiment, appreciation, purpose, will. Comte sees law manifested throughout the phenomena of the universe, and sees nothing more.

Strange that the present Materialist school sets the belief in law as *contrary to* the belief in a Benevolent and Righteous Spirit, the Cause and Ruler of the Universe, when it may be shown that it would be contrary to benevolence and righteousness to influence otherwise than by law! If by God we mean a Wise and Benevolent Spirit, the thought and will of that Spirit would be law. We find that *that* exists which *would* exist if such a Spirit existed. Why are we to disbelieve it?

We see ground for believing, as above said, that a law is nothing else than a thought of God.

Without this staff, we cannot conceive how man can walk with brave and willing spirit through life's difficult and dangerous paths. With it, we can conceive him thanking God even for his mistakes, from which he learns "*right*" for his kind. Life can have no real peace without this belief, viz., that

---

11. Pantheism equates the universe with God, a concept distinct from, though often confused with, that of immanence. The latter, which holds that God is present in but not identical with all things, has appeared in Christian writings from the earliest centuries. As a Platonist, Nightingale felt that God was not only immanent but also transcended the universe. This concept of God as both immanent and transcendent is found in the *Bhagavad Gita* (The Song Celestial), the Hindu scripture that became one of Nightingale's favorite works, as seen in the following passage:

My Being—
Creating all, sustaining all—still dwells
Outside of all!
         See! as the shoreless airs
Move in the measureless space, but are not space,
         . . . .
So all things are in Me, but are not I. (Book Nine, vv. 4–6)

the law, of which the phenomena of the universe are a manifestation, is itself a manifestation of the existence of omnipotent right. All other peace can be only insensibility towards the sin and suffering of our kind.

This dreary rationalism, it is said, strips the universe of the presence of God, and causes it to be inhabited only by His laws.

But what is the difference between God and His laws? His laws are, after all, only the expression of His thoughts. If thought is invariable in Him, so must His laws be also invariable. But we have got into our heads that law is some mysterious chain, which God creates and then leaves—a machinery like the watch, which the maker manufactures, and then sends to a distance out of his own hands. If, however, it is correct to define law as but the unvarying thought of God, law is the continuous manifestation of God's presence—not a reason for believing him absent.

Great confusion arises from our using the same word law in two totally distinct senses, viz., as the cause and the effect. It is said that to "*explain away*" everything by law is to enable us to do without a God.

But law is no explanation of anything; law is simply a generalization, a category of facts; law is neither a cause, nor a reason, nor a power, nor a coercive force; it is nothing but a general formula, a statistical table. Law brings us continually back to God instead of carrying us away from him. To say that a stone must fall *because* of the law of attraction, is but saying that one stone must fall *because* another does, or because the earth tends to fall towards the sun. The *law* of gravitation is merely a general formula, embracing all these facts.

So Quetelet makes his computations that so many people will commit suicide, that so many widowers will marry three times; and we call it, and justly (supposing the computation correct), a law, and then, with our vague ideas that a law is a coercive force, we cry, "Oh! how horrid—then there is a law which compels so many people to commit suicide in a twelve month." But the law, which is merely a *statistical table*, has no *power* to make people commit suicide. So you might as well say that Newton's law has the power to make the stone fall as Quetelet's table to make the people commit suicide. Newton's law is nothing but the statistics of gravitation, it has no power whatever.

Let us get rid of the idea of power from law altogether. Call law tabulation of facts, expression of facts, or what you will; anything rather than suppose that it either explains or compels.

Law, indeed, in the first meaning which we have been discussing, carries us back to another kind of law, a first cause, a conscious intelligent will. If law is in itself no cause, it must bring us back to the cause of law. If law has no power in itself, it must be the expression of a will or power, mental, not physical; and thus laws are only the expressions of the thoughts of God.

Law is, 1st, a general formula, expressing, not explaining facts which co-exist invariably with definite circumstances; 2nd, an intention, or will, in a conscious intelligent being, divine or human, for some uniform co-existence or secession.

All calculation, all foresight, becomes impossible, if we admit no law or preordination, no inevitable and unalterable connexion of facts. If "the Father of lights, with whom is no variableness nor shadow of turning," governs the world, how can phenomena, which are but the manifestations of His thought, be variable and indefinite?

But the conscientious unbelievers of the present day say, that, when all is said and done, and the whole of the faculties exercised, &c., all that we can discern with these faculties is the law of nature.

Comte says, law explains how all modes of existence are what they are. Is there not an absurdity in saying that all we can discern is that whatever *is, is* according to law? For is it not our experience of law that it *always* springs from a will, from a purpose?

If we went to some new country and found a law in operation, but could have no information, no trace of the person who willed, who purposed in that law, we should nevertheless feel an entire certainty, a consciousness that will and purpose had existed in regard to that law.

When we discern a law of nature, we can generally at the same time trace *purpose* in it; is it, then, philosophical or reasonable to say, "We can know nothing as to whether there is or has been a will, a purposer;" we having so much experience that where there is a law and purpose, there is will and a purposer? In the laws of nature we can trace will and purpose of the same kind as exists in man; for instance, love of order, love of beauty, benevolence which wills convenience, ease, comfort.

Mankind has been jarred by circumstances unsuited to right constitution, right development, right exercise of the nature. The thinking part of mankind has been irritated and disgusted by dogmatic assertion of superstitious notions. A revulsion takes place. Many thinkers say in consequence, "I will do my work and believe nothing but phenomena recognized by my senses." Reason and philosophy are now in arms against superstition and dogmatism rather than in peaceful search after truth.

III

Everything—Nightingale felt—nature, people, their thoughts and actions, indeed entire nations, were subject to law. She had arrived at this conclusion as early as 1849, as evidenced by a letter she wrote to her family from Egypt:

Why is there not national like individual progression? . . . It cannot be a law that all nations shall fall after a certain number of years. God does not work in that sort of way: they must have broken some law of nature which has caused them to fall. But are all nations to sink in that way? . . . Or will a nation find out at last the laws of God by which she may make a steady progression?[12]

At first glance Nightingale might appear to believe in determinism, as she describes a lawful universe with an eternal sequence of cause and effect. Later in the text, however, she explains how the laws give human beings their power to become co-creators with God in the evolutionary process. In her view it is the Divine Spirit acting within humanity that provides the creative insight and the guidance through which the universal laws are discovered and applied for human progress.

*   *   *

The whole state of the universe at this moment is the consequence of the whole state of the universe at every past moment, both as regards its spiritual and its physical laws. God does not will "on Monday it shall rain, on Tuesday the wind shall be East," or "the spring of 1852 shall have three months' drought," by an arbitrary decree. The drought of 1852 is the consequence of His meteorological and other laws which have ruled since eternity; not, as in those noble words, "As it was in the beginning, is now, and ever shall be, world without end," but As it was *without* beginning, is now, and ever shall be.

Now, when we read Dalton's[13] discovery that all is by weight and measure, that the proportions in which bodies combine follow a numerical law, as, for instance, carbon expressed by 6 unites with oxygen expressed by 8, and forms carbonic oxide—it will otherwise unite only with oxygen

---

12. Quoted in Sattin's edition of *Letters from Egypt*, p. 74.
13. John Dalton (1766–1844), English chemist and physicist, was best known for his development of modern atomic theory.

expressed by 16, and form carbonic acid, &c., &c.—when we discover such and similar laws, does it not seem that there must be a spirit of wisdom? God is so accurate, so definite; He knows exactly how long we shall go on in a given way, just as He knows how much of the oxygen will combine with carbon, hydrogen, &c.

I once saw an extraordinary storm on the Nile. The river seemed flowing bottom upwards; the whirlwind of sand from the desert literally covering it, and blowing up in ridges upon it. The Israelites might have almost passed upon dry land. Our eyes, mouths, and ears were filled with sand, and it was impossible to drink, for, instead of water from the river, we drew up sand. To try to stand against the wind was useless. Presently five vessels floated past us, keel uppermost, and we saw a little whirlpool of oranges, the unfortunate passengers having broken open the cabin in their efforts to escape. At 3 p.m. it became quite dark, and the waves were like a moderate sea in the Channel. The Arabs thought that the day of judgement was at hand, and were quite helpless.

Now, we know that there was not one molecule of sand or water in that confused whirlwind, which was there by chance, which had not a sufficient cause, so to speak, for occupying the place which it did, which was not rigorously where it ought to be, according to the laws or uniform rules of God.

"No atom of this turbulence fulfills

A vague and unnecessitated task,

Or acts but as it must or ought to act."

In other words, a natural philosopher, who knew the acting forces and the properties of the atoms acted upon, would demonstrate that each atom acted with precision in the way it ought to act, and could not act otherwise than as it did.

In the terrible convulsions which have shaken Europe, have upset empires and annihilated liberty, there has not been one single action, one single word, one single thought, or will, or passion, in the destroyers or the victims, which was not the infallible sequence of its antecedent, which had not uniformly its allotted succession or coexistence in this moral whirlwind. An intellect which could appreciate the acting forces and the character of the nations acted upon could have demonstrated like a Q.E.D.[14] the results.

14. "Quod erat demonstrandum," "that which was to be demonstrated" (used at the end of mathematical proofs).

IV

As religion was subjected to increasing scrutiny from historians and scientists in the nineteenth century, the authenticity of miracles as related in the Scriptures and those described by the Church became a subject of much debate. The question was twofold: whether those who had witnessed the miracles were reliable sources, and whether miracles were possible in a universe governed by natural law. Defenders of the faith held that miracles, particularly those of the Scriptures, proved the veracity of the Christian revelation. Thus to disprove the miracles would be to destroy the very foundations of faith.

Because Nightingale held that the will of God was expressed in the form of universal and invariable laws, she logically concluded that miracles—violations or interruptions of law—can have no place in an ordered universe. She may owe something of her views on miracles to the philosopher Baruch Spinoza (1632–1677), whose writings had gained some popularity in Victorian England through the influence of German intellectualism. J. A. Froude, who later published Nightingale's articles in *Fraser's Magazine*, had written an essay on Spinoza for the *Oxford and Cambridge Review* in 1847; George Eliot had undertaken a translation of Spinoza's *Tractatus Theologico-politicus*[15] in 1849, which contains a discussion of miracles. As will be seen below, the tone of Nightingale's argument against miracles is similar to that of Spinoza, who asserted that "nature cannot be contravened, but that she preserves a fixed and immutable order," and that "God's nature and existence, and consequently His providence cannot be known from miracles, but that they can be all much better perceived from the fixed and immutable order of nature."[16]

Nightingale would also certainly have been familiar with David Hume's (1711–1776) *Enquiries Concerning Human Understanding*, in which he argued against miracles, describing them as a "violation of the laws of nature."[17] In her own discussion, she reiterates his sentiment

---

15. *Life of George Eliot*, pp. 103, 121. Eliot had also translated David Friedrich Strauss's *Das Leben Jesu*, in which Strauss asserted that "where a [biblical] narrative runs contrary to the laws of nature, it must be regarded as unhistorical" (Horton Harris, *David Friedrich Strauss and His Theology*, p. 42).

16. *Tractatus Theologico-politicus*, VI, in *The Chief Works of Benedict de Spinoza*.

17. Hume, *Enquiries Concerning Human Understanding and Concerning the Principles of Morals*, Sect. X, pt. I.

that "a miracle can never be proved, so as to be the foundation of religion."[18]

Contrary to the ideas expressed by Spinoza and Hume (and later Nightingale), the English theologian William Paley (1743–1805) believed that a Supreme Being *could* interrupt the order he had appointed: "In a word, once believe that there is a God, and miracles are not incredible."[19] Paley's *A View of the Evidences of Christianity* (1794) became a bulwark of the Anglican Church, and remained a required textbook at Cambridge until 1920.

The debate continued in the Victorian era with Oxford Movement leader John Henry Newman's essays, "The Miracles of Scripture" (1825–26) and "The Miracles of Early Ecclesiastical History" (1842–43), in which he maintained that miracles were consistent with what we know of God's character. The universe, he posited, functioned in accordance with two systems—physical and moral—of which the moral was superior. Miracles wrought by God for an "important moral end" were thus beyond the action of the laws of nature.[20]

Inspired by the writings of Schleiermacher,[21] some in the Broad Church sought to emphasize the Church's moral teachings rather than relying on miracles to justify the faith. In his *Lampeter Theology* (1856), Rowland Williams stated in regard to Jesus' miracles that "we should lay more stress on the moral significance and beneficence than on the mere element of power."[22] Others, like Baden Powell, professor of geometry at Oxford, went still further, as would Nightingale, attempting to disprove miracles entirely. In *The Order of Nature* (1854) (and later in *Essays and Reviews*), Powell discounted traditional views of miracles as incompatible with his belief in an "invariable universal system of physical order and law."[23] He refuted Paley's and Newman's arguments that revelation is in itself a miracle, contending that "a purely *spiritual* revelation . . . stands on quite different grounds from the idea of *physical* interruption."[24] Miracles might be considered as part of the Gospel but were not proof of it, nor was the Christian faith dependent on the belief in miracles.

18. *Enquiries Concerning Human Understanding*, sect. X, pt. II.
19. *A View of the Evidences of Christianity*, p. 14.
20. "The Miracles of Scripture," p. 18.
21. See Keith Clements, *Friedrich Schleiermacher: Pioneer of Modern Theology*, pp. 118–120, 180–184.
22. *Lampeter Theology Exemplified in Extracts from the Vice-Principal's Lectures, Letters, and Sermons*, p. 46.
23. *The Order of Nature: considered in reference to the claims of Revelation*, p. 247.
24. *The Order of Nature*, p. 279.

Based on a firm belief in the operation of immutable law, Nightingale's arguments against miracles are similar to those of Powell, whom she quotes in *Suggestions for Thought*. Powell's book may have been an importance reference for her as it contains a historical survey of natural philosophy, in which he discusses the impact on religion made by the theories of Bacon, Hume, Laplace, and Comte—all of whom Nightingale considers in *Suggestions for Thought*. Nightingale had corresponded with Powell as early as 1846.[25]

Nightingale's own discussion of miracles in *Suggestions for Thought* may have influenced Benjamin Jowett, who in 1870 was planning to write an essay for a proposed second volume to *Essays and Reviews*, in which he was to discuss the "Reign of Law" and the "impossibility of basing religion on miracles"[26]—precisely the topics addressed by Nightingale ten years previously. He once admitted to her: "I often steal from you."[27]

Despite the arguments proposed by rationalists and the Broad Church, miracles remained an important "proof" of Christianity for Protestants and Catholics alike. J. B. Mozley, a Professor of Divinity at Oxford, maintained in his *Eight Lectures on Miracles* (1865), which reached its fifth edition in 1880, that miracles were necessary as the "guarantee and voucher" of the revelation, distinguishing revelations as true communications from God. Likewise, the first Vatican Council, held in 1869–70, concluded:

If anyone should say that no miracles are possible; and that, accordingly, all narratives about them, even those contained in the Sacred Scriptures, must be rejected as myths or fables; or that miracles can never be known with certitude; or that the divine origin of the Christian religion cannot be rightly proved from them, let him be cast out [*anathema est*].[28]

✳   ✳   ✳

Generally, as the belief in miracles decreases, God dies out. At first, as is very natural, while the laws of God are little, or not at all, understood, people are expecting and finding miracles every day, and see God in them. The Saints lived in a perpetual expectation of a miracle; they speak to God,

25. *Calendar of Letters*, 2.A4,266.
26. Hinchliff, *Benjamin Jowett and the Christian Religion*, p. 108.
27. 28 February 1871, BM Add MSS 45783.f236. Quoted in Vicinus and Nergaard, *Ever Yours, Florence Nightingale*, p. 300.
28. Broderick, ed., *Documents of Vatican Council I: 1869–1870*, p. 50.

He hears and answers; and the state of such persons is truer than the state of the assertors of law is now. Trust in the God who will work a miracle in answer to their prayers, veneration for the God who works the miracle, thankfulness, love to Him for having worked one (though *we* may feel we could not love a God who did work miracles), are truer feelings, juster appreciations of Him, than the appreciation given by the "positive" school of the present day. Alas! that, as the belief in miracles dies out, *God dies out also*.

All religions have been hitherto founded on miracle—on the breaking of law. The present is an attempt to preach religion founded on "law,"—to make God's law His Gospel—His "good news" to man.

Had it not been for the miracles and resurrection of Christ, would the Christian religion have been founded? Would the Mahometan religion have been founded without the miracles of Mahomet?[29] Would the pure, devoted and beautiful life of Christ, His doctrines and teaching have laid the corner stone for Christian religion without His resurrection?

No, this is the first attempt to found a religion upon "law." The Christian doctrines [i.e., without the belief in miracles] would never have founded the Christian religion.

Much attention has been excited, both in devotion and derision, by the Rimini miracle. The beauty of the picture which people call the "winking madonna," and which was 40 years in that small church unobserved, is striking; the expression of purity, holiness, devotion, and melancholy in those up-turned eyes exceeds that of any Madonna, excepting, perhaps, the Dresden Raphael.

But the decaying faith of the town has revived; the besetting sin, swearing, has disappeared, and many conversions have taken place. "It may be the effect of color" has been said, but is it not equally God's way of calling and awakening souls that He, after a lapse of 40 years, should cause the effect to be seen with such results? must we not look with deep reverence on the instrument through which he has worked such a change?

The most striking part of this story is the state of the people which it shows. The picture had been there 40 years, and had remained unnoticed, the "purity, holiness, and devotion" said nothing to them; the beauty of virtue had no effect. *This* did not appear to them to be God speaking to

29. In fact, Islam was founded without the aid of miracles other than that of the Qur'an itself. Despite Muhammad's insistence on his mortal nature (Qur'an 17: 93), apocryphal tales of his miracles developed as early as the Prophet's own lifetime. In his *View of the Evidences of Christianity*, William Paley actually derides Islam for its lack of a true miraculous tradition (pt. 2, ch. 9).

them; but is most affecting how ready they were to listen directly, as soon as they thought that they received God's communication in His "winking" at them. They did not see God in the expression of "purity and holiness," but they saw Him when the picture shut its eyes. God, acting by a law of goodness and righteousness which *never* fails, is really more worthy of reverence than God "winking" at us occasionally, or turning water into wine or into blood, or anything else. It is a most curious fact that a picture making faces should have cured swearing, and a most touching one, that the swearers should have been so willing to listen as soon as they could hear. But that which it tells most loudly is, that this people must be raised and educated till they can hear God's voice in His law of perfect righteousness, hear it in everything—that "still small voice," rather than hear it only in a "*tour de force.*"

People think that they hear God's voice in a miracle now and then; they don't think they hear it in the daily and everlasting expression of His goodness, in the beauty of holiness, in His laws, which are never broken; this *is* very remarkable.

But it is alarming to think how completely we are destitute of the first principles of knowledge with regard to God's nature and His plans with men, His manner of acting. As, till Bacon's time, people were ignorant of the first principle of philosophy,[30] we want a Bacon for the science of God. The crane on Cologne cathedral stands there a monument of man's ignorance of the ways of God. It was taken down, and there was a thunderstorm. They thought God was offended and put it up again.

But, it is said, it is only the most ignorant who have so absurd a superstition as this.

Is it a whit more absurd than the expecting an "answer to prayer," which is expecting that God will alter his laws, His *good* laws, in conformity with our advice—and this when all is as certain as an eclipse? If we prayed that the eclipse set down in our almanacs should not take place, would this be more absurd than praying that one of God's *moral* laws should be altered? Is the crane at Cologne a whit more absurd than the theory of forgiveness and absolution?

People are terrified at the idea of a religion without miracles, and belief

30. Francis Bacon (1561–1626), British statesman and philosopher of science, introduced the idea of science being a collective and systematic enterprise, and developed the first comprehensive theory of induction (reasoning by generalization from previously collected data). Nightingale's scientific methodology was essentially Baconian. She analyzed the disease and mortality rates in different locations and types of settings, and drew her conclusions as to the nature of God's laws regarding health. In the above passage she certainly meant that before Bacon's time people were ignorant of the first principle of *scientific* philosophy.

in miracles certainly makes some happy. It has a cheerful effect to be expecting an interposition every day; but what a lowering of the conception of God!

In all physical things God's law is invariable. We know that if we eat nightshade we shall perish. We take means that our children shall not eat nightshade; we dig it out of our gardens. We don't pray that it may *not* take effect.

We know that certain organizations in certain circumstances will become criminal. The law is invariable. Why do we not take means as in the former case? Why do we, instead of this, think that God will alter his righteous law, his invariable law,—by the invariableness only of which we can learn,—for our prayer?

Without the belief in miracles, in prayer, in a man-God, it is said, we can never have that fervent conviction which Saint Teresa had.[31]

We open a book of science, and we read of a God all order and beauty and goodness, and He excites no feeling. We open the life of St. Teresa, and we find a God all injustice and disorder, and we find her in a rapture about Him. The God of law is always speaking to us—always saying what is wise and good. The God of St. Teresa speaks to her sometimes, and says something which is often foolish and not good. Curious indeed, that, while the God of science never appears to have excited any feeling, the other God has excited so much! May we not hope that the day is coming when we shall feel as much, yea, a great deal more for our God than she did for her's?

Our creed may be felt a dull one by those who have been used to be kept alive by the belief of past miracles, and, in some sort, to look for present ones—since they expect their prayers for restoration of health, for rain or fair, to be answered.

Mankind, however, are not *now* much kept alive by belief in miracles. St. Teresa believed, with her whole soul, the miracles which she relates. But do the many congregations which listen on the appointed day to what was said by Balaam's ass really believe that it spoke? Or, when the same congregation pray for fine weather or for rain, is there a real expectation that any effect from these prayers will result? Is there much vitality in the forms of prayer by law appointed? The religion of the Church of England is mainly now the religion of order, decency, respect. It is probably much better than none; but of how much more is not humanity capable!

Religion now tells of an occasional miracle, meaning an occasional

31. See Chapter 1, p. 12 and n. 10.

effect produced by the immediate will of God. We believe *all* successions, all co-existences to be, in this sense, miraculous. We believe there is no reason, no cause for *any* succession, *any* co-existence other than the will of God.

The beliefs of man have come from the assertions of individuals of their own feelings. The multitude has been led by those who felt fervently. These feelings have been stereotyped, and have been held, after all feeling had departed from the words and practices which once betokened feeling.

Remember these words, "Lo, it is I, be not afraid." Some great artist should paint a series of pictures, where man is passing through sorrow, and God says, "It is I, be not afraid;" where he is passing through sin, even through sin,—yes, *most* through sin, and God says, "It is I, be not afraid." God is so much more there than "walking on the sea," which is, after all, very paltry. Raphael paints Him performing the miracle of the fish, and makes him so divine that we lose sight of the absurd nature of the miracle. But, if he had painted him saying to man in a state of sin and degradation, "It is I, be not afraid," how much more divine!

People make such a point of having the evidence of eye-witnesses to a miracle. But here we have the evidence of St. Teresa that she saw two little devils round a priest's neck. We have the evidence of St. Paul that he saw a light in the sky, and heard a voice. We are as certain of their honesty, we are as certain that they believed it, when they said they saw the devils and the light, as I am that I believe it when I say I see an ink-stand on the table. There is no more ground for suspecting imposture in the case of St. Paul than in that of St. Teresa; but that the devils were not there, and that the voice was not there, we are equally certain. Therefore, what is the "evidence" of an "eye-witness?" Wherever miracles have been believed, they have been seen. We feel as sure that St. Teresa believed she saw the miracle as that she did not see it. There is no difference in our certainty.*

V

Nightingale elaborates here on an idea that was put forward in the first chapter: that if God acts "on a principle" or "according to a rule," then divine forgiveness is impossible. Because mankind learns the laws of

*Baden Powell truly says, Testimony is but "as a second-hand assurance; a blind guide that can avail nothing against reason."

We agree also with Pattison, that "evidences do not constitute theology." [See the Introduction to this volume for discussion of Baden Powell and Mark Pattison.]

God through trial and error and by experiencing the consequences of various courses of action, forgiving the suffering caused by a mistake would actually be cruel, Nightingale believes, for it would impede the development and maturation of humanity. The story of the penitent thief who was crucified next to Jesus, so often used as an example of God's forgiveness, she dismisses as irrelevant:

> It is very evident that the man was very far from being all evil. The very high state of spiritual perception necessary to believe in Christ's kingdom at a moment when his nearest friends considered their hopes blasted and his kingdom destroyed; to pray not for life, not for being saved from the cross, but only for moral salvation, shows that he was already very far on the road to happiness. As far then as he was right he will enjoy happiness, identical with the right. *In his wrong*, not *for* his wrong, he will suffer till his evil becomes all good. But to obtain happiness complete, eternal, while there are any of God's laws unknown, or unobserved by us, is an impossibility.[32]

Nightingale returns to this idea—the futility of trying to propitiate a lawful God—throughout her work, particularly in the sections on sin and evil and on prayer.

*   *   *

The time is coming when, more and more, others as well as ourselves, will discern the little dependence to be placed on supernatural revelation; consequently, let us search to the utmost the *real* grounds man will have for a religion when the unreal grounds crumble away beneath him. The divinities of Greece and Rome, how powerful they were! But they are laid low. Hardly a trace of belief in them remains. The belief in all supernatural foundation for religion will give way in like manner. Many ideas in the present theology are more opposed to natural feeling than those which prompted the worship of some of the pagan deities. *E.g.*, law is *traceable* in all existence, in history of every kind, history of successive generations, of their opinions, their characters, their actions. In vain, then, should we expect the doctrines of particular providence and of forgiveness of sins, to retain their hold on our belief. Yet these doctrines are the staples of religion, as now believed, or as taken for granted. Law is *traceable, i.e.*, glimpses of it have been *traced*. When law was traced in astronomy and geology, Genesis

---

32. *Suggestions for Thought*, vol. 1, p. 150.

ceased to be authority in those sciences. When law is traced in the history of events, and in moral philosophy, Christ will no longer be considered as supernatural authority, speaking, as He does, of providential interference and forgiveness of sins. And when this day comes, where will be our religion? Religion *might* be more felt, more comprehended, infinitely more influential on life than it ever has been.

It is said that Christ is God. But there is wanted a higher God than Christ, a higher God than even Christ's God. Certainly Christ believed that he could work miracles. Can we believe that such would be a God whom we can feel veneration for, whom we can trust in? The God of law is surely a much higher God than this. The God who works miracles is not the highest. We want the *Most* High.

God's plan is to teach all by invariableness. See how opposed this is to miracles, which teach by variableness! And how are we ever to learn when we cannot be sure of what is coming?

When Christ says, "faith shall remove mountains," he appears to think that if you can but believe it, God will break a law. For to remove a mountain in the way He implies would be to break a law. No doubt the expression was used merely as a strong and startling one. But he would not be a wise man who would wish to break a law of God. He would be the wise man who believes that God will *never* break His laws, not that, if *he* believes that God will, He will. Certainly Christ's was not the God of Law.

But some think that the theory of omnipotent and implacable *law* is not more satisfactory than that of benevolent caprice, the recognized form of Deity. They think this a miserable world. If they are to be miserable, it does not signify to them whether they are miserable in consequence of such misery being the law, or whether they are miserable in consequence of such misery being the caprice of the Superior Being. On the contrary, they would rather it were caprice, because then there might be some hope that the caprice might change, whereas, if it were the law, there would be no hope.

But it makes some difference *what* the Being is from whom emanates the law. If the law emanates from Juggernaut, certainly we would rather have caprice. But, if the law springs from wisdom and goodness, had we not rather have invariable law?

If it is wisdom and goodness that I and all the world should work out perfection, and that perfection cannot be worked out without ignorance and mistake and misery, does it not *then* make a difference to us whether we are governed by law or caprice?

We must know the purpose of the artist, before we can appreciate his performance. If human physical ease were God's purpose, He has failed. Is it proved that He has failed, if His purpose is a habitation on the heavenly bodies for the exercise of goodness, benevolence, wisdom, righteousness in man? for the attainment of perfection by imperfection, of knowledge by ignorance?

Is it not of the very highest importance to find out God's character?* Is not God's character our only dependence for a future state? We seem to think *that* a very poor dependence. But if we could make out God's character from the things we see, should we not be able to make out the things we do not see from God's character? I do not feel the slightest doubt from knowing your character that you will not commit a murder. Cannot I feel the same certainty about God? What is the difference between His and your committing a murder? and what is killing one of us but committing a murder? Does the fact of being possessed of Omnipotence justify it? And why should we suspect *Him* of it?

What is meant when you say the word "forgiveness?" People forgive, but how do they do it? Probably they think of something else. If a man knocks me down, and if I feel that he is the greatest sufferer, because he is further from the way of right or happiness by the act of knocking down than I by the fact of being knocked down, and if I feel that by the laws of the universe he could not have done otherwise than he did, I can—not forgive, but—feel no resentment, for he could not have done otherwise. But if I am told that I am to forgive another because God forgives me, what have I to do? I must think that that man has been very wrong; but then I have been very wrong, too, against God, and He has forgiven me; and if I don't forgive this man, perhaps another time God will not forgive me. What does that mean? It means that I think of something else, of God's wrath and my sins against Him, and so I forget what has been done against me. Can any other meaning be attached to the theory of forgiveness?

Belief in universal law leaves the word *forgiveness* without a meaning. If it is true that, whatever man has thought or felt, all his inclinations, whatever has been his will, have arisen in accordance with law which it was

*"Theology" is said by Pattison to be—"1. The speculative habit which transports the mind into another world. 2. An ethical principle regulative of our conduct in this world." Is not theology rather the knowledge of God's character? Is it not a curious thing to leave out all mention of God in that which is, if anything, nothing but the science of God, and to call such science a "speculative habit?" One might as well call the study of astronomy a "speculative habit." God, whom perhaps we may call the only reality, is the subject, of all others, which we shake all belief in, as a reality, by this kind of speaking.

not in his possibility to annul or to alter, it must be unmeaning to ask God to forgive a past, which arose in accordance with His law, or man to forgive what was inevitable. Anger, indignation against the individual sinner, must be untrue feeling in whatever being it exists.

Forgiveness is certainly a step beyond revenge. In the first state of society, it was considered right to revenge our injuries; in the next state, it was considered right to forgive them; though how this is done we do not know. Still, this is a step in advance. This is already a "future state" to the first. In the next "future state" it will be considered that there is nothing to forgive; and that will be a doctrine as much higher and truer than this of forgiveness, as this of forgiveness is higher than that of revenge; but the philosophy of the will must be first understood.

With regard to forgiveness in the Creator, the theory is no more intelligible. "God cannot forgive" is true, and it is curious how people lay hold of a little bit of a truth. *God cannot forgive;* His laws have assigned consequents entirely definite to every antecedent. Do we pray that he will prevent oxygen from uniting with hydrogen in the proportion of eight to one to form water? Neither can we pray that he will alter the laws of perfect goodness and wisdom with regard to spiritual things. *He* would not be perfect goodness and wisdom if He did. But the theory of forgiveness, as the Anglican Church holds it, is besides, a confused one. What sign have we that we are forgiven? How do we know when we are forgiven? The Roman Catholic is more sensible, who takes his beads and says so many paternosters for every sin, as his confessor orders. "We don't know how to pray," he says, "therefore we take our Saviour's form of prayer, which is much better than anything we can say, and we take each sin in succession, and say, 'Forgive us our trespasses, &c.;' and then say, 'that sin is forgiven,' now on to the next." Is not this the theory of the rosary when used "in union with" our Saviour's sufferings? The Roman Catholic does think of his sins enough to tell them each and individually to a priest, who is the intermediary, and who tells him whether he is sorry enough, and, if he is, gives him absolution, thought what takes place when we are absolved we do not know. But Protestants have such a "slovenly unhandsome" way of doing the business. We will not even take the trouble of enumerating our sins, but we say, in order to save ourselves that trouble, "We have done those things which we ought not to have done," in order to include everything; and then "*bang* comes the absolution," without more ado. But what takes place when we are forgiven? Is it a change in God or in man? What is it? We know no more than if you were speaking Chinese.

"Taking a clergyman's duty," the very words are significant, it is a *duty* to pray to God; and when the clergyman wants to do something else, he gets somebody to "take his duty." We do it in the most lazy way we can. We get one man to say it all for us (while we sit by),—to say that we have done everything wrong.

The doctrine of forgiveness, though an advance upon that of revenge, is still, therefore, the great mistake with regard to God's character, the character of the Perfect, of perfect wisdom and goodness.

The Spirit of Right could not forgive without an absurdity. Will God make that which has been, not to have been? alter that which is past? The prayer would be impertinent, if it were not absurd. For it is asking the Spirit of Right to produce a contradiction, to be in opposition to Himself. But He is always the same; "yesterday, to-day, and forever."

* * *

As with so many of the issues Nightingale addressed in *Suggestions for Thought*, the idea of "forgiveness" was one she had contemplated years before. In a letter to her father, she explained that forgiveness is only a step in the evolution of human consciousness. Forgiveness pre-supposes a sense of personal injury. When one comes to the realization that the universe operates according to law, there will be no feeling of being victimized and thus no need for forgiveness. God, whose under-standing is complete, *cannot* forgive as He is impossible to offend:

I have often wondered how Christ could teach that prayer, "And forgive us our trespasses, as we forgive those who trespass against us"—when certainly that is not what we wish but a great deal more. But that prayer it now seems to me, was the most practical embodying of a great philosophical truth, perhaps the only intelligible popular form of it. For, first we must begin by making the effort to forgive others ourselves, before we can possibly realize that God *can* extend forgiveness to us. Next, we must have learned to forgive others sponta-neously before we can believe in the *spontaneous* forgiveness of God and what is the next step which takes place in ourselves? Why, we begin to see (after having practiced these two long enough) that we have no business with forgiveness, for we had no business to feel the angry revengeful feelings . . . the renuncia-tion of feelings in *ourselves* is what we agreed to call "forgiveness" & till we see this, see, i.e. that *forgiving* is *giving up* an evil passion in ourselves, we cannot realize the great Truth, that there is *no* forgiveness in God—forgiveness being essentially the property of a fallible being, not of God, (tho' the Collect does say so) who has nothing to do with it. This Truth now appears, not as the opposite proposition to Christ's prayer, but as its natural and direct *consequence* at which indeed we could not have arrived without praying long and often (till it became a practice) that prayer. And as Religion is the popular practical form of Philosophy,—so that prayer Christ saw to be the only popular practical ladder to this great idea of the nature of God.[33]

33. Letter to W.E.N., 12 October 1848, Claydon Collection (*Calendar of Letters* 2.E2,421).

3. On God's Law and Human Will

In accordance with God's law, human consciousness is tending to become what God's consciousness is—to become one with the consciousness of God.

I

To give man a will, an identity, a freedom of his own—and yet so to arrange that his will shall become freely one with the will of God, is the problem of human existence—for the will of God being the will of perfect love and wisdom, is the only will that can lead to perfect happiness. The will of man, therefore, in order to attain happiness, must be the same as the will of God.

Can this problem be solved otherwise than by giving man such a nature, and such circumstances acting upon his nature, as shall induce it to be his will to do that which is for the happiness of mankind, in which his own is included?

We admit that His happiness and ours consists in the same thing—that our thoughts, feelings, &c., can only be happy in as far as they are like His, which are truth.

The operation of God's will in law appears to be that in human nature, through the operation of law, there shall be such desire for, or satisfaction in, right—that in successive time mankind will discover how to attain progress in right for mankind. Man will within certain limits become the creator of the human constitution, or, more properly speaking, will modify it for its proper objects—man will determine within certain limits the circumstances of human life—determine them with the purpose of progress in righteous existence for man. *Thus* the Almighty and Perfect affords assistance to the imperfect and ignorant.

II

As mentioned previously, Nightingale was able to convince government officials and policy makers of the need for public health reform through her use of the newly developed tool of statistical analysis. She demonstrated the relationship between unsanitary conditions and disease: when sanitary reforms were instituted in the military hospital at Scutari during the Crimean War, the mortality rate dropped from an incredible 42.7 percent to 2.2 percent. Disease is caused by unsanitary conditions, she was convinced; and because the universe is lawful, humanity has the power to change these conditions and thus prevent disease.

Nightingale's emphasis on the wholeness of the individual and her belief in a lawful universe convinced her that mental, as well as physical phenomena, were regulated by law. In this area she drew heavily on the work of Adolphe Quetelet, who demonstrated yearly regularities in the age-specific crime rates for both men and women, in various countries, and in different social groups.[1] The theoretical foundations of his "moral statistics," or "social physics," which he developed in the early 1830s, were that (a) social phenomena, in general, are regular and their empirical regularities can be discovered through the application of statistical techniques; and (b) these regularities have causes: the social conditions at different times and in different places. Casting doubt on free will and individual responsibility for crime, Quetelet's work provided a basis for arguing that better social legislation would improve social conditions, thus lowering the crime rate.

Although Quetelet's work was respected by many scholars, it was criticized by others. Helen Walker, the historian of statistics, wrote that Quetelet's contemporaries

scoffed at him because he dared to suggest that a man's moral qualities might be measured by his actions and his intellectual vigor by his productions. They called him a materialist because he deduced from statistical documents facts which ran counter to the current theory of free-will. . . . He was convinced that the measure-

1. Quetelet, who learned probability theory from Laplace, published widely and carried on a voluminous correspondence with a multitude of prominent scholars (see discussion in the Introduction, pp. xi–xii). Material from his early articles on "social physics" was published in 1835 in a book entitled *Sur l'homme et la développement de ses facultés: physique sociale*. He personally presented to Nightingale a revised and expanded version of this work which was published in 1869.

ment of mental and moral traits waited only upon the collection of sufficient and trustworthy data, and that when such measurement was feasible, it would be found that the distributions of these traits conformed to the normal law.[2]

Quetelet's research was consistent with and supported Nightingale's spiritual philosophy. Far from demeaning human nature, making it a puppet on the strings of circumstances, she felt that the statistical view of human behavior ennobled and empowered the human race. If "mental and moral traits" are, as Quetelet theorized, a function of the circumstances of the individual, then mankind has the power to create the circumstances which would incline the heart to "keep God's laws aright."

*   *   *

Let us understand that *our power* arises from God's invariableness.

We can never too forcibly remember that, because what has been in the past could not have been otherwise, it by no means follows that we are powerless over the present and future.

If we can and *if* we will alter those specific conditions out of which past evil arose, it certainly *will not* recur.

Granted that certain circumstances invariably involve one definite constitution of the human physical being, whence springs the whole capability of that being—granted that circumstances invariably affect definitely this being, so that all he is results from law—is this necessity? is this making him a machine? is it not accordance with right? is it not putting power into his hands? For he has capability to find out how to bring about right physical being—right circumstances in which to live.

While Director-General Andrew Smith[3] was in power, it was "the gate to the kingdom" of the Army Medical Department to say that yellow fever was an "inscrutable dispensation," and that nothing could be done to avert it.

Many have believed that cholera was traceable to no other origin than the direct will of superhuman power that it should exist; and the means attempted to prevent it were prayer, which, it was hoped, would influence God's will, or some changing of circumstances totally irrelevant to the case.

2. Walker, *Studies in the History of the Statistical Method*, p. 41.

3. Dr. Andrew Smith (1797–1872), Director-General of the Army Medical Department in 1853–58, authorized Nightingale's nursing expedition to the Crimea. During the Crimean War he was subjected to much criticism from the press and from Nightingale herself.

This divine will is now shown, by experience and observation, to be that wherever certain physical conditions (such as want of draining, of cleanliness, &c.) exist, cholera, in epidemic years, will exist; that these physical conditions ceasing to exist, cholera will cease to exist.[4]

Buckle says, "In India slavery,—abject, eternal slavery,—was the natural state of the great body of the people, the state to which they were doomed by physical laws utterly impossible to resist."[5]

Granted, so long as circumstances rule man. But God's laws will teach man to rule *circumstances.*

"Thou shalt not kill" is said to be God's law; but this is not God's law, for men *do* kill; while God's law is never broken. Men *do* kill, and if they *could* not kill, there would indeed be no "liberty." This is Moses' law, not God's law.

Again, Quetelet shows that not only such a per-centage of men *will* kill in a year, but such a per-centage out of this per-centage will use such a weapon, such a per-centage will use poison, &c. This does not show that God decrees that a certain number of murders shall be committed every year, but that certain states of mind, and certain circumstances co-existing, murder will be committed.

Again, it appears that boys between the ages of 15 and 20, although they constitute only one-tenth of the population, afford an amount of crime which constitutes no less than one-fourth of the total crime committed in that population.

But these are the announcements of the statistician, not laws of God.

It is the result of God's law that, given such organizations and such circumstances, given such a state of society, such a number of murderers will there be; and further, such an amount of evil will be entailed on society, teaching it the truth about crime.

It is the result of God's law that, given such a state of society, and such of education, such an amount of boy-crime will take place.

But what is this but to say that we must bring about *another* state of society and of education?

If, indeed, we were to see a spotless and virtuous generation of youth growing out of the present education and state of society, then indeed we

4. Nightingale never accepted the theory that germs are the causative agents of disease. Rather, she felt that disease is a reparative process instituted by nature to eliminate from the body toxins absorbed from a polluted environment (see *Notes on Nursing*, pp. 7–12, 94).

5. William Henry Buckle (see Chapter 2, note 9).

should be at a loss to conclude anything else but that this God has "withdrawn himself to a distance," and has laid down no *law* at all.

✳   ✳   ✳

The theory that human behavior is a function of circumstances was put to the test by Nightingale during the Crimean War, with respect to the drinking problem among the soldiers at the Scutari Hospital. They complained that they had nothing else to do in their spare time but drink, and they had plenty of money for it because they distrusted the official means of sending paychecks home. The officers did nothing; they looked down on the soldiers as hopeless drunks and let many die from the poisonous liquor.

Trying to remedy the situation, Nightingale made it a practice to stay in her room four afternoons a month to receive the money of any soldier in the hospital who wanted to send it back to his family. The money went to her uncle Samuel Smith, who bought postal orders which he sent to the various addresses. With the aid of private funds, she was instrumental in organizing a reading room and two recreation rooms. Nightingale herself supplied the newspapers and writing material. Woodham-Smith describes the effects Nightingale's reforms had on the common soldier:

"The men," she [Nightingale] wrote, "sat there reading and writing their letters, and the Library of the British Museum could not have presented a more silent or orderly scene." The officers had told her that the men would steal the notepaper and sell it for drink, but this never occurred.

By the spring of 1856, four schools, conducted by professional schoolmasters, had been opened. "The lectures," she wrote, "were crowded to excess so that the men would take the door off the hut to hear. . . . A more orderly population than that of the whole Command of Scutari in 1855–1856, though increased by the whole of the Cavalry being sent down there for winter quarters, it is impossible to conceive."

It was an astonishing achievement, and during the winter of 1855–56 the picture of the British soldier as a drunken intractable brute faded away never to return. "She taught," said an eye-witness, "officers and officials to treat the soldiers as Christian men."[6]

According to Nightingale's philosophy, all phenomena—even undesirable ones like murder—arise in accordance with law. As she ex-

6. Woodham-Smith, *Florence Nightingale*, pp. 167–168.

plains below, God decrees the laws that determine human action but not the specific action itself.

*   *   *

If a law existed in any mind that a certain number of murders should be committed every year, we may safely say such a mind is not good or wise.

The idea of God either under a "*necessity*" to make such a law, or making it of his own "free *will*," is obviously a contradiction in itself, if by God we mean a spirit of wisdom and goodness.

No being that could be called *good* would bring other beings into existence under such conditions as these; viz. of living under a law which compels men to be in such a state of mind as that they *must* commit murder. It is quite another thing to say that there is a being, whose thought is the progress of imperfect natures towards perfection; such progress being worked out through the exercise of faculties existing and regulated in accordance with his law or plan—the consequence of such law or plan being that a number of men of a certain organization, and in certain circumstances, will have the inclination to commit murder. Such are the conditions of human nature: viz. that a certain number of persons *are* so circumstanced that it is their will to commit murder. This is a fact. No one will deny it.

To say that they are *necessitated* to commit murder would be again self-contradiction; for it is their determined will, the fulfillment of that *strong inclination* without which no man ever committed murder.

The practical result of such a belief as that above stated would not be to induce us to cease the struggle to prevent or to reform sin; but the very reverse.

In proportion as a mind feels some horror at the idea of a fellow-creature murdered, and *much more* horror at the idea of the state of mind in which a man is who commits murder; such a mind will be urged to ask itself, Can I do anything to alter this state of things consequent upon which this number of murders is committed? Can I,—directly or indirectly, at once or in course of time, individually, or with the help of others,—raise the human mind to such a state as will prevent or lessen murder?

We who are moralizing have no distinct impression of what the previous life is of any one who has committed murder. Can we doubt that, if we had, if we understood the framework of the human spirit,—in other words, its organization,—if we could trace the various influences affecting a man from his birth to the commission of such a crime, we should perceive when and how the inclination to commit it might have been prevented, the mind opened to better influences?

Such would be the practical power of this belief, when united with any strong horror of sin,—with any strong conviction of the power of man to raise man out of it,—that it would be an *imperative* call upon the human heart and understanding so to improve man's circumstances as to "incline his heart to keep God's law" aright.

With regard to the horrors described in the pages of human history, let us listen to them well. It is the Eternal voice,—"*Not so*, my Children." "*Not so*" we hear also repeated in every cholera, massacre, vice, degeneration. Man usually replies to it by prayer, (if he replies at all,) prayer for the removal of the evil. And the Eternal voice answers again, *Not so*. Cease to spend yourselves in vain. What is this buzz of purposeless talk from thousands of re-unions of such talent as *might redeem* mankind? What is this rattle,—ceaseless in your cities yet purposeless for man's divine nature,— when such a purpose waits to be fulfilled? Will you stand by, or pursue these inane follies while the divine nature of MAN is being murdered or while he is murdering himself? Or, as inanely, will you betake yourselves to prayers for the salvation of man to Another, whose express plan it is that it shall be your own noble work? The poisoned, the paralysed nature cannot help *itself*. Man must rise up and save.

*   *   *

Although Nightingale believed that human progress requires a change in the consciousness of the race as a whole, she wrote that certain individuals, or "saviours," must serve as facilitators:

The world cannot be saved, except through saviours, at present.

Now what are the saviours to do? Not to do anything *instead of* man. Still it is not intended that every man shall learn all the laws of God for himself. In astronomy, Copernicus, Galileo, Kepler, Newton, Laplace, Herschel, and a long line of saviours, we may call them, if we will,— discoverers they are more generally called,—have saved the race from intellectual error, by finding out several of the laws of God.

In the same way, there may be, there must be saviours from social, from moral error. Most people have not learnt any lesson from life at all— suffer as they may, they learn nothing, they would alter nothing—if they began life over again they would live exactly the same life as before. When they begin the new life in another world, they would do exactly the same thing, and they must, till somebody comes to help them. And not only individuals, but nations learn nothing. A man once said to me, "Oh! if I were to begin again, how different I would be." But we very rarely hear this; on the contrary, we very often hear people say, "I would have every moment of my life over again," and they think it pretty and grateful to God to say so. For such there can be no heaven; in fact it will not be there for them to have till saviours come to help them. This *is* "eternal death."

We sometimes hear of men "having given a colour to their age." Now, if the colour is a right colour, those men are saviours.

People think that the world is in the mud, and that it must stay there. *We* think it is in the mud too, but we are sure it is not to remain there.

III

> Concerned that her idea of fixed and immutable laws might raise questions concerning predestination and free will, Nightingale felt it necessary to clarify her views, contrasting them with those of the Protestant reformer John Calvin. Calvin believed that God had pre-ordained some individuals to eternal life and others to eternal damnation; Nightingale believed such a position to be inconsistent with God's benevolent nature. God does not decree individual actions, thoughts or emotions, but only the laws by which they are governed. God's laws serve as the means by which all of mankind is ultimately to become one with God. Thus man is predestinate inasfar as he is subject to divine law. Mankind is not powerless to bring about his own salvation, as Calvin had maintained, but has the capacity to discover the laws of God that would lead all into a "state of grace."

*   *   *

All existence depends at each moment on God's will. He wills not special *decrees*, but certain uniformities or constant relations of succession and of co-existence, which we call *laws*, and which we might call habits or rules of nature. These we can ultimately refer only to God's will, explain only by saying that they are His thoughts.

All these relations are merely means and inducements supplied by God to enable man to attain his proper development, which is to be one with God—("I and my Father are one"), to have the same object, the same thoughts, feelings, wishes. The Son is to have everything that the Father has, not as a gift, but to be obtained by mankind for mankind. In this way man will partake even the omnipotence of God, when he desires nothing but what God desires. Then will he, by the laws of God, accomplish everything that he desires; and what can God do more?

The proposition that the smallest circumstance comes to us from the will of God is true in this sense. A man is and does what he is and does, because it is the will of God that certain definite perceptions, thought, emotions, volitions, shall succeed or co-exist with certain organizations and circumstances. It is not true in the sense that each particular perception, thought, emotion, volition, is caused directly by the decree of God that so it shall be. In the former sense, it is our business to discover, to desire and to attain the circumstances and organizations which produce the right volitions, &c., that is, those which are one with God's. This discovery we are intended to make by experience, not our own individual experience alone, but the collective experience of all mankind.

If it were not invariable that definite characters flow from definite circumstances (and in many cases we can actually predict it), man would be acting at random; he would never discover with certainty, either for himself or others, what course would lead to right. God does not thus deal with us.

In one sense indeed we *are* predestinate. We see a ragged creature, brought up in Field Lane or Saffron Hill, at the "thieves' kitchen and seminary for the teaching of that art to children," and we truly say that he is "predestinate to sin and death." We see the child of Lois and Eunice brought up amid great objects "unspotted from the world," and we can truly say he is predestinate to grace and salvation.

All children, however, brought up in St. Giles's[7] do not grow up thieves; all who are carefully and piously educated, as we but too well know, do not grow up good men. Is there something besides the inevitable action of circumstances, as it is called?

These exceptions are also the subjects of law; the effects are also traceable to some circumstances, unknown to us, but which could have no other effects.

---

7. The parish of St. Giles-in-the-Fields in Soho was notorious for its poverty and squalor and was vividly described in Charles Dickens's novels. In the 1840s the London Statistical Society determined that more than forty individuals lived in each of the five-room houses on Church Lane in that area.

Then, it is said, this is implying an unbroken chain, held in the hands of God, from the first beginning of things, upon which is strung every event, act, feeling, thought, will of a man's life; effect following cause, as link follows link, immutable, pre-ordinate.

The nature, however, it is said, remains under the free will of a responsible agent.

This is to say, in fact, that God interferes with some things and not with others, that He, by an act of arbitrary will, lays down certain landmarks, and leaves man to live as he likes during the meantime. How do you explain "insulated phenomena"? Can such be? Phenomena are only the manifestation of God's thoughts. Insulated phenomena are as much as to say that God thinks at one time and not at another.

This, it is said, is a far more dangerous pre-destinarianism than that of Calvin.

It is true, we are predestinarians, each in his own sense. The difference between this predestination and that of Calvin is, that we believe all are predestinate ultimately to the happiness of the Creator himself: any idea of punishment, not intended to improve the creature, being inconsistent with a Being of perfect goodness. We believe cordially that the laws of God are so arranged as to flagellate us with our sins, and to attract us with their opposites, so as, at an appointed time, (appointed, not by *decree*, which is an express volition of God, but by *law*,) to bring us, i.e., all, into a state of grace, as it is called.

Then it is said, we have nothing to do but to lie still and wait till "*the laws*" whip us into goodness. Free will, adieu!

But what is meant by free will? A power to will whatever I please? Certainly, you may will whatever you please; but the very question is, what you will please? What you will please is decided by your nature. Will is only the emanation of the being. It is as impossible that a being should will contrary to itself, as that a flint should emit carbonic acid gas, or charcoal silicine acid.

We object to the character of *free* will being solely appropriated by the opinions it is used to express, which suppose will to be unregulated by law—not to exist in definite relation—to have no regulation, no origin, other than the determination of the mind in which it exists.

It cannot be said that the will is *not free*, because it accords with law. We understand absence of freedom to be impediment, through will and power in *another* nature, to a man following the inclinations of his own. Does the supposition that will accords with law imply that any external will prevents a man willing in accordance with his nature? By no means. No external will is supposed to decree that an individual nature shall be in a state from which some definite volition will follow. The supposition is, that each volition consists with, is simultaneous with, or successive to, a definite state of the nature. Yet we should not use the phrase *free will* to express this conception, though, supposing it true, we consider the will free, in the accepted meaning of *free*. To say that the will is free, would but give a part of an explanation of what we have to express.

The Calvinists tacitly admit that free grace implies irresponsibility. If we miserable worms are to be scaling heaven when and how we please, where would be our sense of reverence and awe when we look up to God, of humiliation and utter helplessness when we look down upon ourselves? they ask. God alone can call us, of His free grace and election, according to His purpose before the foundation of the world.

This predestinarianism reduces us to the level of animals. A man is no better than a dog to which its master all at once begins to teach tricks.

If this be so in partial pre-ordination, often called election, observe that, on the contrary, universal (not partial) pre-ordination is the only system of things by which any power at all can be given us from above. Without the laws of God, which pre-ordain the minutest connexion (we will not say, consequence) of things, how could man have any power at all for carrying his will into effect?

But it is said his will is, according to this doctrine, the offspring of his nature, which is the offspring of previous circumstances; therefore his will itself is not free.

The word "freedom," however, is improperly used in this case. For "freedom" should we not rather substitute the word "power"? And this power to put his will into effect must be wholly dependent upon law. If circumstances were to have sometimes one consequence and sometimes another, how could we calculate so as to produce any effect which we desire?

IV

In her letter to John Stuart Mill asking him to read *Suggestions for Thought*, Nightingale wrote that she had been greatly influenced by his book *A System of Logic* (1843), "especially as regards 'Law,' 'Free Will' and 'Necessity.' "[8] In the last section of the book, "On the Logic of the Moral Sciences," Mill coined the term "ethology" for the science of the formation of character. He wrote that, although the human mind functions according to law (that is, volitions and actions are the effects of causes), a human being can choose to be determined by some causes as opposed to others. Thus one has, to some extent, the freedom to alter one's character.

Developing this idea within her own spiritual philosophy, Nightingale wrote that the only means of attaining ultimate well-being is to align the personal will with the will of God. It is not the freedom of choice which is the important element, but the power to create those causes which will make the human character reflect the Divine.

* * *

It is often said that the nature or mode of operation of the will is beyond the human understanding. We believe that there are questions on that subject beyond our reach. But that uniform relations exist between *volitions* and *sensations, thoughts,* and *emotions,* and between those states of mind and the constitution and circumstances of the individuals in whom they exist, appears evident from experience.

If a certain state of mind produces a wrong will (whatever this thing, called the will, may be); if another certain state of mind produces a right will—surely it is of as much essential immediate vital practical importance to each and to every one of us to know—1. Whether there are laws; 2. What these laws, if any, are (which bring about those distinctive states of mind)— as it is to know whether one kind of berry, when eaten, produces a healthy state of body, another causes sickness or death.

Belladonna poisons the body; bread feeds it. The question whether there are poisons and foods constant in their operation, if it had not been answered centuries ago, would be of *vital physical* importance to us. No one in a healthy sane state knowingly takes belladonna for food or bread for poison. Here constant laws are admitted to be in operation, and no one dreams of his "free will" being thereby limited or destroyed. No one says that, because he cannot feed himself with belladonna, nor poison himself with bread, therefore he is not a free agent.

8. Letter to J. S. Mill, 5 September 1860; quoted in "Florence Nightingale as a Leader in the Religious and Civic Thought of Her Time," p. 78.

But the other question—the moral question—remains still in the uttermost confusion.

Not only is it still a question whether there are any laws at all, constant in their operation, of which certain states of mind are the result—of which states of mind, again, a right or a wrong will is the result—not only are we almost entirely ignorant what these laws are—that is, *what* does poison the mind, *what* does feed it—but there is a perfect outcry against even making the inquiry because it "implies a limit" to our "free will!"

Suppose a man's will to depend on a self-determining power. It has been maintained that this is so, to the extent that any man could, if he pleased, resolve any morning never to do wrong again, and *keep* his resolution by force of such self-determining power. Believing that experience contradicts such a supposition, we also consider it a most dangerous one, inasmuch as the tendency of such belief is to turn the mind from the possible, the necessary, the essential means of attaining right will in man.

Nor would it seem right, or analogous to anything we know, that one accustoming himself to do wrong for years should be as able by a single resolve to secure a righteous will, as one who had been striving for the good for years. A man who has taken opium for months does not conceive that he could resolve to do away with all its consequences at once, and be to-morrow morning in the same state as if he had drunk nothing but pure water.

Let us suppose that uniform relations exist between human will and the constitution and circumstances of the individual in whom it exists. On this supposition we have power to determine the will aright, if we use appropriate existing means. Man has power over unborn generations, over the will of his contemporaries, over his own will, if he used the appropriate means. He has power to affect the constitution and the circumstances which affect the will. To explain how, by what means he may possess himself of this power, how to exercise it aright, would include the whole compass of human knowledge, all available for this object.

Sanitary science is showing how we may affect the constitution of the living and of future lives. In one direction, sanitary science is understood to apply to the physical nature; but each part of man's nature affects every other. Moreover, there is a sanitary science essential to each of man's faculties and functions. For each there is an appropriate state and operation—in other words, a healthy state; and there is a science discoverable as to how, by what means to bring about that appropriate state.

Not only have we the power to modify existing constitutions—we have power to regulate circumstances favourably to individual idiosyncratic constitutions (meaning by *favourably* so as to induce a right state of the nature—*i.e.*, of the will.)

The source of will being sensation, thought, emotion, states of mind which vary with definite conditions—by bringing about the appropriate conditions, man may attain right will.

What power will the righteous man desire in regard to the will? Is it the power to will either right or wrong? Will he not rather desire a state in which it will be in his nature to will right; in which to will wrong will be impossible to him? A mother who deserves the name does not contemplate a state of will as even possible in which it should be at her "choice" to mangle, ill-treat, and starve her baby, *or* to nurse, love, and tend it. It is impossible to her to will the first. It is in her nature to will only the second.

What is the Creator's own character? He cannot choose between good and evil. *Cannot* is indeed a wrong word, as implying that He would if He could. But to suppose the Creator willing evil, is a contradiction. In this sense God himself has no free will. The nature of the Spirit of Goodness is turned unvaryingly to good. What may we suppose is His object with His creatures? Not that they should attain a free will to choose between good and evil, but such a nature as that nothing but good will attract, no evil will tempt it. Surely if you were bringing up a child, you would not wish to educate it to make a free choice whether it will be a murderer or not, but to be one to whom murder is impossible. When, therefore, our natures, by the Creator's laws, have been brought into that state that we not only know that right is happiness, but feel it,—know how "to incline our hearts to keep this law,"[9] we shall not will to commit evil,—not because we shall have acquired what is called "free will" to make a choice between good and evil, but because we shall no longer be capable of willing evil. To approximate to such a state, law affords man means—the means, namely, that he may learn by experience how to modify constitution and circumstances, how to adapt circumstances to constitution, so that the nature, the will, will be right.

Often we do calculate, and are deceived! Not, however, because the law has failed, but because some other laws, unknown to us, are concerned, which, when we know them, will ensure our calculation, based upon

9. From the responses to the Ten Commandments in the Book of Common Prayer.

absolute fore-knowledge that effects can never vary nor be uncertain or indefinite. When we know all God's laws we shall be omnipotent like Him, for we shall desire nothing but what He wills.

This is a quibble upon the word omnipotence, it be said. Killing every wish that cannot be satisfied is not omnipotence. Supposing we know and can employ all God's laws, it does not follow that we shall not desire something which those laws will not give us. It is an old story: the child who cried for the moon.

But what is God's omnipotence? To satisfy our idea of omnipotence, must it be able to do everything which tongue can speak—to effect a contradiction—to effect that a thing should be and not be at the same time—that a thing should have been and yet not have been—to make the past not be—to make injustice justice, cruelty mercy, wrong right? Is all this necessary to satisfy the condition that "all things are possible with God?"

If God repented, or wished to make the past not be, He would not be God. He would have made a mistake. A Being who could wish to effect a contradiction or an absurdity would not be God; and that Being who could wish to make wrong right, we are quite sure, would not be God, but devil. Is it necessary to make God able to do that which he does not wish, to satisfy our idea of omnipotence? If not, the same definition, which answers our conception of God's omnipotence, will also satisfy it in man's case.

When man knows all God's laws he will perceive the full beauty of them; it will be impossible for him to wish one to be altered, for he will see that if one were other than it is, man could not attain the full happiness prepared for him; it will be impossible for him to wish other than what God wishes, because he will see the perfection of it. Is not this the meaning of what St. John says, "We shall be like Him, for we shall see Him as He is." Then shall we no longer say, "Father, not my will, but Thine be done," but "Father, Thy will is mine;" and therefore all that we desire will be done. Do we wish for a greater extension of omnipotence than this?

V

According to the Athanasian Creed, incorporated in the Book of Common Prayer, ". . . they that have done good shall go into life everlasting, and they that have done evil into everlasting fire." This clause and scriptural passages that speak of eternal damnation sparked much controversy in Nightingale's day, in large part a consequence of the writings of Frederick Denison Maurice. His discussion "On Eternal Life and Eternal Death" in *Theological Essays* (1853) led to his dismissal as professor of theology at King's College. Rejecting literal interpretations of the creed and scripture, Maurice asserted that:

eternal punishment is the punishment of being without the knowledge of God, who is love, and of Jesus who has manifested it; even as eternal life is declared to be the having the knowledge of God and of Jesus Christ."[10]

Nightingale was well aware of the controversy surrounding Maurice's assertions. His sister Mary was a member of the governing committee of the Institution for the Care of Sick Gentlewomen in Distressed Circumstances, where Nightingale served as superintendent. Nightingale was so troubled by Maurice's forced resignation that she threatened to leave the Church of England, and even thought of resigning her position at the Institution, which had strong ties with the Church.[11]

Eternal damnation was as central a tenet of the Church as was that of the Trinity. In response to remarks made in *Essays and Reviews*, more than 10,000 clergy signed a declaration upholding the doctrine of the "punishment of the wicked."[12] Refuting it was thus clearly not a matter to be taken lightly, as Maurice indicated:

... theologians have in our age become entirely positive and dogmatic upon this subject; that upon it can they brook no doubt or diversity of opinion; that in fact, they hold that man is as much bound to say "I believe in the endless punishment of the greater portion of mankind" as "I believe in God the Father, in God the Son, and in God the Holy Ghost."[13]

The debate over eternal damnation did not end with Maurice's dismissal, but continued into the 1870s when unsuccessful attempts were made to exclude the Athanasian Creed from the Book of Common Prayer.[14]

Nightingale herself expressed disbelief in eternal punishment as early

10. Maurice, *Theological Essays*, p. 307.
11. *Calendar of Letters*, 3.F4,763.
12. Altholz, "The Mind of Victorian Orthodoxy," p. 191; Chadwick, *Victorian Church*, vol. 2., p. 84.
13. *Theological Essays*, p. 315.
14. Wheeler, *Death and the Future Life in Victorian Literature and Theology*, pp. 192ff.

as 1846, as evidenced by a letter to her aunt, Hannah Nicholson.[15] Because she believed in a benevolent God whose purpose it is to lead all of humanity to perfection by means of His laws, she found the belief in eternal damnation to be repellent. Since human will is determined by divine law, God could not justly punish mankind. Man's suffering is rather the result of his ignorance of the consequences of his actions:

Man is "predoomed to misery" only on his way to something else, and in order to give him something else.[16]

If human actions are determined in accordance with divine law, what then is the difference between right and wrong? Nightingale felt that right, or happiness, is being in accordance with the will of God, or, as Maurice indicated, having the knowledge of God. The very pain of our "punishment," which is the disharmony between the human and divine will, is the motivation that impels us to change our behavior.

*   *   *

It is urged that the whole doctrine of reward and punishment is by this theory swept away, for how can the human being, whose will is formed for him, be, in any way, with justice, a subject of reward or punishment? he only does what he is made to do. The Creator has made his creatures what they are. How can He punish or reward them for it?

As we arrive at a truer conception of God's moral government, we shall find reason to modify the meaning of various words used in describing it. We find that *punishment*, if the word be used in the sense of suffering or privation consequent on sin or ignorance, does exist in God's moral government, and we see it to be right, because its effect will be sooner or later to induce mankind to remedy the evils which incur it. But eternal punishment, or vicarious punishment would be the satisfaction only of revenge, not of justice. It seems strange that under *any* interpretation of the rule of the Being whom we call perfect, it should be supposed that an eternity of suffering is destined for beings whom it cannot benefit, since their future knows no hope or possibility of amelioration. It seems strange to suppose

15. *Calendar of Letters*, 2.A3,265.
16. *Suggestions for Thought*, vol. 1, p. 150.

that He whom we call love, righteousness, could only forego the satisfaction He would have exacted for sin, by substituting an innocent sufferer.*

Admitting, however, that law so operates that our passage to truth and right is through the evils incident upon ignorance, it is evident that no punishment but that which is remedial, is consistent with justice.

Punishment, in the sense of suffering consequent on wrong-doing, and designed by the eternal laws to drive the criminal to another course, we can understand, and such punishment we cannot wish to have remitted. But punishment, when there is no further power of amendment, there is hardly a human being who would wish to inflict.

Let us give up altogether the ideas and the words implying reward and punishment. In sermons and pious books, "sinful pleasures" are generally treated as the natural desire of the human heart. "The heart is desperately wicked and deceitful above all things." These words are quoted as reason for the belief. By the *nature* of man, the constitution of man, we mean the state which *befits*, which is appropriate to man according to the laws of his being—and thus understood, the proper, the healthy nature of man is averse to sin. It "thirsts after righteousness." In sickness, a man loses what is called his natural appetite. So it is with a corrupt mind, or a mind not constituted, or not developed so as to feel the *natural* wants of the human mind. Wrong is invariable suffering or privation of man's proper *well-being*. Right is invariably well-being, or the road to it.

This eternal immutable (we will not say connexion, but) *identity* of right and happiness, of wrong and misery, is very commonly lost sight of, and it is thought that our nature tempts us to sin; that sin would be pleasant, if only God, by His arbitrary will, had not decreed that we should be burnt for it.

How can there be any right and wrong if there is no "free will?" it is asked.

It is a law of God that a certain wind acting upon a tooth in a certain state, tooth-ache shall be the consequences. Because you could not help it, does that tooth-ache cease to pain? Do you say, it was not my fault; I will not care about it? On the contrary, the very pain is the motive which

---

*Our surprise is, however, diminished by the reflection, that frequently, as the popular theology repeats the words "eternal damnation" in its services, the idea does not dwell in the understanding, in the heart, or even in the imagination. To hear the concluding quaver of a chant rest on those horrible words, sufficiently brings home to us how little they affect their hearers.

compels you to get rid of it and to avoid it in future. Right and wrong are as immutable as pain and ease, the one to produce happiness, the other misery. And we talk of "God making allowances for the frailty of His creatures," "not being prone to mark what they do amiss," "having mercy on his erring children." This mercy would be the height of cruelty. As long as His laws have not inflicted evil consequences on our sin and ignorance till no vestige of either is left in us, mercy means to leave us in sin and consequently in misery.

To escape God's justice our "Common Prayer" appeals incessantly to His "*mercy*." But "mercy" is a word without meaning, in the perfection of divine government. If the consequences attached by His law to sin, for the purpose of weaning us from it, are too severe, to inflict them would be injustice, to relieve us from them would be an act of simple justice, not of "justice tempered with mercy;" if they are not too severe, their remission would be an injurious concession, equally derogatory to a perfect rule. Mercy for *past* sin would mean a change of mind in God.

The pre-ordination of inevitable consequences is essential. Without this, right would produce sometimes happiness, sometimes misery, calculation would be at fault, motive would be wanting. There would be nothing to incline the will more to good than to evil, without the pre-ordained connexion between good and happiness, evil and misery.

Can a doctrine be immoral where goodness *is* happiness, not connected with or the cause of it, but identical with it?—where wickedness is misery? The other doctrine says that there is always a hope that God will forgive,—that we may sin and yet escape the punishment. But the only happiness worth having is God's happiness; and the divine happiness, that happiness which we are *all* to share, is not the consequence of goodness; it is goodness. But where happiness is made to depend upon some change of mind in God, and not in man,—where, as in the case of the dying but repentant sinner, God is supposed to forgive, that is, to change His mind towards him, and bestow happiness as an arbitrary gift,—can there exist than this any more immoral doctrine? God *gives* us nothing. We are to work out a happiness, like His, in ourselves, in accordance with His laws.

4. On Sin and Evil

That they should sit down satisfied with saying that "evil is a mystery," that "God's ways are inscrutable," appears no less extraordinary, when we consider that evil is only the essential ignorance of man's beginning, and that God has constituted us expressly to discover all His thoughts.

I

WHAT was God's purpose in creating us? Some say He created us for His glory, to honour and to serve Him. Others say that this is ascribing a motive, viz. vanity, to God—which we should not dare to assign to a good man—in whom all regard for his own glory is supposed to be extinguished. Some think that God created man for happiness. Others say that they see so much suffering—that either happiness is not God's purpose, or if it is, He fails in it.

The argument that suffering brings forth greater general happiness than there could be without suffering, is met by the objection, that God is, in that case, wanting either in omnipotence or in benevolence. If He is benevolent, He will desire to avoid all suffering; if He is omnipotent, He will be able to do it, *i.e.*, to secure the highest good without the suffering.

God's thought is truth, God's feeling is happiness. God's will is wisdom. How will he cause other beings to partake in these things is the question. Will His plan be to effect that they shall, by His decree, think His thought, feel His feeling, do His work? to oblige each thought, feeling, act, to be what it is. Will He make a creature which cannot go wrong; instinct, or the voice of God, always telling it what to do, and being always obeyed?

Such beings do exist (but we call them beasts), which never make a mistake and never improve, and are incapable, as far as we know, of happiness, that is, of God's happiness.

The problem, then, to solve appears to be how shall our thought, feeling, act, be like His, yet not through the exercise of His powers, but of ours, not by His will obliging each to be what it is, but by our own springing from our own nature. How shall God, in other words, communicate His own happiness, the essential of which is activity, without depriving our happiness of its essential, *our* activity?

Would it not be a contradiction to suppose that Perfect Benevolence would will to other beings a nature less perfect than His own, less adapted to goodness and happiness? But it would also be a contradiction to suppose Him willing another perfection, (since, essentially, perfection is one), or willing an eternal *imperfect*, with such degree of value as could be imparted to it by its being a passive recipient from God. Avoiding these contradictions, may we not, without contradiction or absurdity, pronounce that the Perfect would will limits to His own perfect nature, according to a law of right; these limits to be enlarged by the individual and collective exercise of mankind? That this is actually the fact cannot with truth be denied. There are laws with respect to the material nature, which material nature is the limit to the Divine nature. According as that material nature *is* after a certain type, and is exercised in a certain mode, the divine nature becomes more and more apparent. This rests upon fact—and could, otherwise, the expectation be realized that the Perfect would will His own nature to other than himself? Could the expectation be, other wise, realized that, through exercise, not as passive recipients, God's benefits should be attained by men? And let us observe how exercise, for each and for all, would thus be called forth. Man thus becomes, in some sort, the creator of man.

One and another cause of suffering disappears from time to time by the exercise of man's capabilities. We can see glimpses of how others might disappear, if he used these capabilities differently from what he has done. Great increase of enjoyment has been opened in certain directions by exercise of man's capabilities, and here too we have glimpses into immeasurable enjoyment attainable by man.

Do not such observations lead to the conjecture that the higher will intends man to work the way from suffering into happiness by exercise of capability?

The capability of each individual when born, the development and improvement of this capability, are obviously left in large measure to mankind. In no other race is there this dependence on the race itself. Do not these considerations point (shall we say empirically?) to the suggestion that man shall perfectionize man?

We who have been called upon to walk through varying scenes of life, to see the pure and the noble, to see the debased, can tell that mankind, in general, little conceive the misery of iniquity, but still less the heaven within a man's nature, from which he is in banishment, because his capabilities are not exercised. Mankind must unite to organize life, so as to exercise these capabilities. Meantime, the divine nature "descends into hell."

II

If God is benevolent, omnipotent and just, then how do we account for the existence of evil? This is the dilemma of *theodicy*, in which Nightingale was keenly interested.[1] Every belief system, if it is to be complete, must address the existence of evil in the world. Nightingale attempted to resolve this issue, as have philosophers and religious teachers throughout human history. During her journey through Egypt in 1850, she pondered the question of evil when she came upon a temple scene depicting King Rameses II being crowned by the gods Horus and Seth:

It was the Great Ramesses crowned by the good and the evil principle on either side. What a deep philosophy!—what theory of the world has ever gone farther than this? The evil is not the opposer of the good, but its collaborateur—the left hand of God, as the good is His right. I don't think I ever saw anything which affected me much more than this (3000 years ago)—the king at his entrance into life is initiated into the belief that what we call the evil was the giver of life and power as well as the good . . .

The old Egyptians believed that out of good came forth evil, and out of evil came forth good; or as I should translate it, out of the well ordered comes forth the inharmonious, the passionate; and out of disorder again order; and both are a benefit.[2]

Nightingale's explanation of evil is consistent with her spiritual philosophy; she is also following a line of thought that appeared early in the Christian tradition. As will be seen from her remarks, her concept of evil bears similarities to those of Meister Eckhart and Giordano Bruno, as well as to some of those of Augustine.

Influenced by the neo-Platonist philosopher Plotinus, Augustine (354–430 A.D.) offered two different explanations for the existence of evil: (a) evil is the privation, corruption, or perversion of Good, which is

---

1. See Introduction, p. xxiv, n. 54.

2. *Letters from Egypt*, p. 96. The 1854 edition of *Letters from Egypt* contains the complete discussion of evil, pp. 128–130. Additional remarks can be found in "Vision of Temples," which was appended to the 1854 edition of *Letters from Egypt*, pp. 328ff.

the ultimate reality;[3] (b) what appears to be evil, from the narrow human perspective, is a necessary element in the wholeness of God's universe.[4] It is the latter solution Nightingale's thinking resembles.

The German mystic Meister Eckhart (whose work was valued highly by Christian von Bunsen[5] and thus perhaps familiar to Nightingale as well) held that evil, that is, the privation of good, is necessary in the divine plan because it impels mankind to strive toward greater goodness. In this sense, sin is attributable to God:

> A good man ought so to conform his will to the divine will that he should will whatever God wills. Since God in some way wills for me to have sinned, I should not will that I had not committed sins; and this is true penitence.[6]

Developing this concept further, the Italian philosopher Giordano Bruno (also a particular interest of Bunsen's) held that evil was necessary for the soul to realize its true nature, which is perfection:

> On the one hand evil is necessary for good, for were the imperfections not felt, there would be no striving after perfection; all defect and sin consist merely in privation, in the non-realization of possible qualities. It would not be well were evil non-existent, for it makes for the necessity of good, since if evil were removed the desire of good would also cease. In its whole life, however, the soul will realize all good, and therefore is only per accidens imperfect.[7]

Nightingale's concepts of sin and evil were also in common with those of Friedrich Schleiermacher, who, as already noted, profoundly influenced the Broad Church movement in England. Schleiermacher attributed sin to divine causality, indicating that God must somehow allow sin to exist, for if He did not permit it, He would most certainly destroy it.[8] Noting the role of sin in the evolution of consciousness, Schleiermacher remarked:

> If sin has a place in our nature, it is so closely connected with everything else that our consciousness cannot be complete until it, too, has really emerged.[9]

3. *City of God*, XII, 6–7.
4. *Confessions* VII, 13.
5. See Introduction.
6. *Meister Eckhart: The Essential Sermons, Commentaries, Treatises, and Defense*, p. 79.
7. J. L. McIntyre, *Giordano Bruno*, p. 314. See also the discussion in the Introduction, p. xxviii.
8. *On Christian Faith*, 79, 1; 80, 2. See the discussion in the Introduction, p. xxii.
9. "Second Sunday after Trinity, 1831," III, 8. Quoted in Karl Barth, *The Theology of Schleiermacher: Lectures at Gottingen, Winter Semester of 1923/24*, p. 44.

In his comparative study *Christianity and Hinduism*, Rowland Williams also pointed to the divine origin of evil: "Since that which we call evil, comes of eternal possibilities, or of necessities conditioned to creation, so it has, in one sense, its root nowhere else than in the mind of the Creator."[10]

Nightingale's concept of sin and evil as developed in *Suggestions for Thought* may be summarized as follows:

a) "The imperfect is the Perfect, limited by material relations or, in other words, that man is God, modified by physical law."[11]

b) To attain happiness and well-being, mankind—through its own efforts—must actualize or "enlarge the limits of" its divine nature. This is God's plan for humanity.

c) Mankind is capable of creating the circumstances which facilitate its evolution to the perfection of God through knowledge of the universal laws.

d) Since humanity must attain this knowledge through trial and error in an eternal developmental process, mistakes will inevitably be made.

e) Sin, evil, and suffering thus arise out of ignorance of both divine law and God's plan for the evolution of humanity.

f) Evil is part of the divine plan because it alerts the human race to its mistakes. Thus without evil the developmental process could not proceed.

*   *   *

What is the origin of evil? the question so often asked. *The wisdom, goodness, and righteousness of the Perfect, the Father,* is the answer; who wills that Man, the son, by the exercise of his nature in accordance with the laws of right, shall rise from ignorance to truth, from the imperfect to the perfect.

If we inquire into God's dealings with His creatures with trust that they will be found to arise from goodness and wisdom (since otherwise they would not be God's dealings), we shall come to this question, May not sin have become introduced into the world from ignorance of one or more of God's laws, sin being something untrue in our feelings, our thoughts, our wills; something unlike the feeling, the thought, the will, of God?

10. *Christianity and Hinduism*, p. 341.
11. *Suggestions for Thought*, vol. I, p. 194.

How can He cause that which is unlike Himself? may be asked.

As an infant stumbles, and the mother sees it better that it should stumble rather than never learn to walk alone, so it may be said that the stumble is ultimately caused by the mother's will; thus the sin may be caused by the will of God the Father, and yet be unlike His own. Now, all sin arises from ignorance of God's laws at some time or in some individual.

From ignorance? it is asked, when "I *knew* it was wrong."

You knew it was wrong to do what you did at a particular time; but there was a time when that in you which led to this sin was called out unknown to you; when there was nothing stronger than it in your character.

With regard to our physical being also, all suffering, all privation of that enjoyment of which man is capable, arises from ignorance of God's laws, either our own ignorance, or that of those who have preceded us.

"Did this man sin, or his parents?"

That question implied a false idea. Sin regards those laws only which concern our spiritual and moral being, that is, our feelings and wills towards God and our fellow creatures. That a man is blind implies some ignorance of physical law, either on his own part or on that of those who preceded him.

Those physical laws may have been disregarded in consequence of something wrong in the spiritual life. Disease in the spiritual being will often lead to indulgence in malpractices in the physical. But the immediate cause of blindness is a physical law. And it is untrue to regard a physical evil as a punishment, that is, an arbitrary infliction for some spiritual evil.

If the question is asked, shall we ever learn all these laws? Do we even know one of them?

In time, that is, in eternity, we shall. God has formed us in the image of himself, and therefore we cannot doubt that man's happiness is to be the same as that of his Father.

We may see into God's plan, and see it to be not only one of entire and perfect goodness and wisdom, but the only one by which man could share in the divine happiness, become individually one with Him in will, yet while doing what God wills, remain an individual will, not a machine, and be for ever advancing to share His power, His wisdom, and love,—the plan which gives us the strongest incitement to try to find out and to do what is right. All this may be proved by the reason, felt by the feeling, and approved by the conscience.

Never let us give our belief unless our reason, feeling, conscience, are all satisfied; even though we cannot satisfy reason, feeling, conscience, by any other belief. Rather let us remain respectfully in doubt. We must not only compare our sources of belief with those of others, but we must compare each of our own sources among themselves. Feeling, if in a healthy state, is as important a source of belief as reason. The phrase *"human reason"* is devoid of sense. Is reason more human than feeling, or less super-human than conscience? Let us listen to them all, for these are the voices God has given to be our guides.

Divine and human nature, understood as far as man *may* understand, will reveal that there is no mystery in the existence of evil. God's laws are ever in activity, ever open for the investigation of mankind. To understand them, and to act in accordance with them, these are our means to turn all evil into good. All existence, except the Perfect, is essentially finite; the Perfect would not be perfect unless He destined the finite to rise to the Infinite. Let us not lament and despise our finiteness, but rejoice to look upon it as the mark of our "high calling" to ascend.

There will be always evil, because there will be always ignorance. But there will not be always masses of evil, lying untouched, unpenetrated by light and wisdom (in as far as man is concerned), except now and then a temporary improvement by *chance*, not after a type and purpose.

Each advance has always brought evil with good, because each advance must, in some degree, be made upon an hypothesis. But mankind, when they work after a type, will, more and more speedily, turn the evil into good. We shall not wish to part with evil in the abstract, when it is understood to spring from ignorance, when all the faculties of all mankind are directed to expect evil from ignorance, and to remedy it. Then, though it will be the essential attendant on the imperfect and finite in its progress towards perfection and infinity (through exercise of mankind, of *each for each* and *for all*), there will be a perpetual and rapid change of evil into good; thence fresh temporary evil, thence fresh permanent good. And so on, through the universe, through eternity; the Perfect assisting, teaching, giving successive revelations to the imperfect, by His laws which furnish means and inducement by which the imperfect may advance towards the Perfect;—thus it has been *without* beginning, is now, and ever shall be.

If we see no evil, the possibility of removing which does not exist in *mankind* (as a whole), why are we to stand wondering that God permits evil? do we want Him to give us no work? or to do our work for us? would that be wisdom, benevolence, love, in Him? Let mankind fulfil its possibilities. That will answer the question; is the existence of evil compatible with the existence of a Being of perfect wisdom and benevolence? When we see a man about to be drowned, saved by the wisdom and kindness of a fellow-creature, we do not *then* say, *can* the Being be benevolent, who allowed man to be liable to be drowned? We admire in Him that He gave the saviour capability for the work of love, that man is saved by the exercise of the capabilities of man, by divine wisdom and love manifested in the "earthly vessel."

God has no mysteries for us, any more than the teacher has who commits a problem to his pupil to be worked out, the which could not benefit him but through the exercise of the pupil's own nature. Thus much we know, viz., that a human being, constituted in a certain manner, and that constitution co-existing with certain circumstances, will manifest those attributes, the manifestation of which is all that we know of the Being whom we call God.

We also know that it is in the power of human beings to affect the constitution and the circumstances of themselves and each other,—that, in some instances known to them, they have power to affect the constitution and the circumstances of themselves, of their children, of their fellow-creatures, *in such a way* as to increase or lessen the manifestation of the divine attributes in them.

It is true that the wrong a man does comes from within; that he must undergo suffering or privation till he is conscious that he is wrong—till that wrong becomes right. Take the case of disease. That disease arose, partly from physical circumstances which concerned the beginning of his existence, partly from those after his birth, before he could have any part in his own destiny; partly from those after he could know what was right, which prevented his knowing how to make his volitions right. It is one thing to know what you ought to do, and another to know how to do it; one thing to know the law, and another to know how to incline your heart to keep that law. But the sick man must be conscious that his physical frame is in a wrong state, must suffer the consequences of its being wrong; perhaps during life, perhaps till it can be put into a right state; and nothing can exempt him from them.

It is, therefore, a true feeling that the wrong, whether physical or spiritual, which a man has within himself, must produce for him suffering, which no one can bear in his stead.

It is said that it is very hard that man must suffer for faults which, according to this theory, he could not avoid.

Hard that man should attain to perfect happiness? Man possesses reason, feeling, conscience, *capable* of unfolding, so as to be one with God, that is, to think His thought, to feel as He feels, to will that His will shall be done, and thus to share His happiness, His power. Is this hard? God, it is true, gave him no instinct *how* to cultivate these capabilities aright. Mankind has to learn by experience, 1st, what are his capabilities? 2nd, what are all the various laws of God concerning them? 3rd, that it is desirable to cultivate these capabilities aright; 4th, which of these laws enable him to do so? 5th, how to keep them? 6th, how to incline himself to keep them. All this man has to learn and to practice before he can be one with God.

But the first man had had no experience. He would be *certain* to be ignorant of most of these laws. It would indeed be *impossible* for him to discover them all. It is impossible for us now. Time is the key to God's thought. It is the *word*. In time God's thought is ever being worked out. Without a constant reference to ever passing time, we *must* misunderstand it. It requires united man in all time to discover all. When we pray to be "kept this day from all sin," to be "delivered from evil," we utter a prayer for that which is impossible.* Unless we have perfect knowledge of every one of these laws, we *must* err. Our prayer is a contradiction. If we were "delivered from evil," the world would be ruined, its only safeguard gone— God's plans are all for eternity.

God has provided that mankind shall attain, therefore, by their own effort to progress towards being as He is and doing as He does.

And if they fail, their will may still be one with His; and this oneness with Him in will shall give comfort where the finiteness of created nature prevents their being and doing as the Infinite.

"Be ye perfect, even as your Father in heaven is perfect." Yet will man never be God, but one with God; and when he suffers, he will yet have joy in feeling "Thy will be done."

III

The doctrine underlying baptism was a point of serious contention among the various factions of the Victorian Church. In accordance with the Thirty-Nine Articles, the High Church maintained that baptism

---

*In the Lord's Prayer, beautiful as it is, there is hardly a word of exact truth. "Our Father which art in heaven." If He is anywhere, He is *everywhere*—not more in heaven than on earth. "Thy will be done in earth as it is in heaven." We do not know whether there is any other place where His will is done more than in this, at present; and, in one sense, His will is always done. "Forgive us our trespasses," when the trespasser in His pioneer, cannot be true. Neither can "deliver us from evil," when He made the evil by His laws on purpose to save us. [Editors' note: the prayer to "be kept this day from all sin" is from the Book of Common Prayer.]

constituted a regeneration or new birth, whereby an individual was accorded remission of original sin, promised forgiveness of sins in the hereafter and was "grafted into the Church."[12] Evangelicals, however, stressed repentance throughout life, and were thus wary of a doctrine that promised saving grace at the beginning of one's life.

Sensing "the imminent peril to all that is dear," Edward Pusey felt compelled to articulate the Tractarian position in his *Scriptural Views of Holy Baptism*, in which he provided a discursive theological argument defending baptismal regeneration, while underscoring the Church's role as the interpreter of Holy Scriptures. F. D. Maurice retorted with a "Letter on Baptism" (later incorporated into *The Kingdom of Christ*, 1838), which cost him the professorship of Political Economy at Oxford at the hand of Pusey. Although Maurice believed that baptism brought man into a state of union with Christ, he declared that it was not a "momentary act," as Pusey had implied, "but a perpetual sacrament."[13]

The debate over baptism intensified as a result of the highly publicized case of George Cornelius Gorham, to which Nightingale directly refers in *Suggestions for Thought*. Over sixty books and pamphlets were written on the case, and *The Spectator*, a weekly news magazine, reported: "Every word of the arguments in the Gorham case, every quotation cited, every explanation offered, were perused by men usually content with police reports."[14]

Gorham's evangelical views of baptism came under scrutiny when he became a candidate for parish priest in the diocese of Exeter. After being interrogated by Henry Phillpotts, Bishop of Exeter, for a total of eight days between December 1847 and March 1848, Gorham's appointment was denied. Maintaining that "regeneration" *might* occur at baptism but was not guaranteed, Gorham appealed his case before the ecclesiastical Court of Arches, which nevertheless concluded that his views were indeed contrary to Church doctrine. The case was brought before the Judicial Committee of the Privy Council, a state rather than Church body, thereby calling into question the very authority of the Church. Nightingale's friend Christian von Bunsen was in attendance on the day in March 1850—over two years after the case began—when the decision was handed down. The committee ruled that Gorham's views were *not* contrary to those of the Church, which had never been

---

12. E. J. Bicknell, *A Theological Introduction to the Thirty-Nine Articles*, p. 368.
13. *The Kingdom of Christ; or Hints to a Quaker*, vol. 1, p. 347.
14. Crowther, *Church Embattled: Religious Controversy in Mid-Victorian England*, p. 18.

clarified in the course of the hearings in any event. The decision caused an immediate outcry from the Tractarians, and many, including Henry Manning, Nightingale's friend, left the Anglican Church and embraced Roman Catholicism.

"The belief in original sin is untenable," Nightingale wrote, "if law is found by experience to operate as we have interpreted it."[15] From her point of view, every human being has an inner divine nature that will be realized through a knowledgeable application of the laws of God. She took the Church to task for not dismissing the whole question of baptismal regeneration, which she regarded as "abominable" and "diabolical" since it implied that God was "the worst of tyrants and murderers," having condemned infants to endless suffering. This was, she wrote, "another superstition about the nature of God unparalleled for its atrocity in any savage tribe."[16]

*   *   *

That a Church which does not call itself inspired, of which Queen Victoria is the head, which embraces nearly all the cultivated men in the kingdom—that this Church should say that it was an open question whether babes who died unbaptized were damned or not—that it did not signify—it might be so—men might believe one or the other, as they chose—is one of the most curious historical phenomena we know.

It pre-supposes such an idea of God—that He should elect a babe from all eternity to everlasting damnation. The Atonement does not give such an idea of Him. A man may dwell upon the justice of God, and then upon His goodness, in finding out this plan of saving us from hell, till he forgets the badness of plunging us into hell. But the doctrine of predestination—viz., that He chooses *for all* eternity a little child for hell—and the Church of England theory that she does not know—she may believe it or not, as she will—does seem unparalleled in the history of belief.

We see no *evidence* that man is created righteous or unrighteous, nor any reason why he *should be* created in one state or the other. The babe enters the world neither in one state nor the other, unless the diabolical doctrine be adopted of "baptismal regeneration." The babe *becomes* the one or the other, according as its thoughts, feelings, character, in short,—are

15. *Suggestions for Thought*, vol. 3, p. 68.
16. *Suggestions for Thought*, vol. 1, p. 214.

developed by its circumstances acting on its organization. If we will, we can, to a certain degree, affect organization, and, when we cannot affect it, adapt circumstances favorably to it. And if mankind at large attain to desiring the right, they will learn more and more to bring about this, viz., that both organization and circumstances shall ensure continual progress, in righteousness, of being and of life.

Can any evil be shown in human life not *more or less* remediable by power, wisdom, and goodness *attainable* by man? Who shall say then what is the evil that is not remediable?

We acknowledge that there are certain laws, the consequence of which is that the child's physical, intellectual, and spiritual nature is affected by the parents. We acknowledge, therefore, that children begin their existence in a certain definite state, which would have been different from what it is, had the parents been different from what they were.

In consequence of the first individuals being ignorant of some of God's laws (which is the natural consequence of its being God's plan that men should learn by experience), the children inherit some deficiency of organization.

The "sins of the fathers are visited upon the children," not only "unto the third and fourth generation," but throughout all generations. This process has been going on as long as man has existed. The laws which influence descent and which concern the well-being of man are almost unknown. Yet each has taken its natural effect since the beginning of the race. It is probable that, knowingly or unknowingly, from self-indulgence or inevitably from the state of society and circumstances, all parents have more or less disregarded the laws for securing a well-constituted nature to their children.

This is not supposing a constant degeneration in the race of mankind; because another process is also going on, a process of regeneration. Man improves by experience. God and the divine spirit in man are ever at work to turn the evil into good.

We may truly say that there is "original sin" in each of us; that is, sin which originated with our first parents, and the effect of which exists in us; we sin because the first man sinned.

*   *   *

In Christian theology, the atonement (lit., "at-one-ment") signifies the reconciliation of man with God through the death of Jesus Christ.

According to the Thirty-Nine Articles, Christ served as a sacrifice "not only for original guilt, but also for all actual sins of men." This idea was generally rejected by both Unitarians and the Broad Church. In his commentary on the *Epistles of St. Paul*, Benjamin Jowett summarily repudiated commonly held notions of the atonement:

> The doctrine of the Atonement has often been explained in a way at which our moral feelings revolt. . . . The only sacrifice, atonement, or satisfaction with which the Christian has to do, is a moral and spiritual one; not the pouring out of blood upon the earth, but the living sacrifice "to do thy will, O God"; in which the believer has part as well as his Lord.[17]

Nightingale too rejected the doctrine of the atonement, believing rather that sin can only be dispelled by the knowledge gained from one's mistakes.

*   *   *

On the doctrine of sin, as held by the church, necessarily follows the atonement. *Unless you say,* "man sins by God's law, and his sin (or ignorance) is to be removed by the increasing knowledge of mankind, which is to be gained by the exercise of their own faculties," you will say, "I sin—I cannot help it—I must have an atonement to save me. Else I am lost." For your very theology teaches you that you must never hope to avoid sinning in this world.

Man had a dim perception of God passing through sin and suffering for man and in man, and also of sacrifice and compensation—though it does seem a curious sort of compensation that His Son should suffer and die because we have offended Him—the whole scheme of grace and redemption appears to be an elaboration of error founded upon some truth. And yet this is believed, and the simple scheme of God's providence men are scandalized at; it is indeed necessary to have a church to keep up all this.

Atonement for sin, by the suffering of One who has not sinned, is a popular feeling at variance with that interpretation of God's thought, to which belief in universal law leads us.

The main principle of God's government thus interpreted is that man shall work out progress in knowledge and righteousness for humanity—shall suffer through his errors, not because God is angry, but because the

---

17. *The Epistles of St. Paul to the Thessalonians, Galatians, Romans*, vol. 2, p. 547.

Spirit of Goodness and Wisdom we name *God* thus conducts us through our work to righteousness, which is our well-being. Man shall not enjoy the high possibilities of his nature, except through the proper exercise of that nature; he is in a state of privation while he knows or seeks it not.

The popular doctrine, on the contrary, is that man can do nothing for himself; yet that God's anger against his sin is such that only by suffering consequent on that sin, can He receive satisfaction, propitiation. Such is God's condemnation of sin, that all who have sinned must have suffered eternally for the satisfaction of God; but that One perfect in righteousness has in another manner offered satisfaction—propitiation for sin—has, in some way incomprehensible to us, made Himself guilty of all sin ever committed, or to be committed, by man, and so suffered as to satisfy the Divine nature, and to save men from the sufferings which would otherwise follow from their sins, provided they believe in the sacrifice thus offered for them.

Such belief, though directly contrary to the conception of the Divine nature and government which we believe to be revealed by law, yet generally accepted as it is, offers much to call forth reflection, and impress the mind, even in those who differ from it. It shows the sense, the feeling concerning moral evil which has existed in the human mind—the increased force of such feeling, since such atonement was conceived necessary and the belief in it accepted.

IV

The Greek mythology was the deification of the powers or laws of nature. The Christian mythology was the deification of the spiritual laws or ways by which communication exists between God and a half-savage, half-corrupted man ("I am the way," Christ says)—a man who fancies to himself God offended with His own creation, and taking His revenge upon it. If Christ were obliged *now* to speak to the judges, magistrates, and staff of our criminal courts, where He heard the word "punishment" used, must He not speak of the mercy of God to those whom He sees condemning criminals, in perfect good faith, to places where they must lose every ray of humanity still shining within them? For is not mercy the only goodness which society can apprehend, while we still conceive the idea of *punishment*, still have the word at all, instead of reformation? A Christ *must* speak of the forgiveness of God: society can conceive of nothing else.

Those who don't believe in reformation, in Sir Joshua Jebb,[18] in Lord Shaftesbury,[19] and the ragged schools,[20] have attributed the same impotence to God. He *can* only hang them, and put chains on their legs, as we do. "The Court feels bound to pass a severe sentence," what does that mean? and the criminal "is imprisoned for eighteen calendar months," what is that for?—merely to keep him out of mischief for that time? or to deter others by terror? or to reform him? We know that the second of these objects is not attained, and the third is not even aimed at. Would it not be better to let him out? But no, "the Court feels bound to pass a severe sentence," and God feels bound to give the sentence "of everlasting chains under darkness." Can He too only punish, instead of reforming? The idea of eternal damnation had its origin amid a society which exercised punishment; and as soon as mankind sees that there is no such word, that reformation is the only word, eternal punishment will disappear out of our religion; everlasting damnation and capital punishment will go out together.

*   *   *

In the previous chapter Nightingale takes the view that, in a lawful universe, criminal behavior is a function of the condition of society; the prevention of crime should thus involve the reform of society rather than the punishment of the individual criminal. Here she calls for reformation again, from a somewhat broader perspective. The essence of her argument is that (a) if all human beings have a divine nature and, according to God's plan, are to attain perfection and (b) if sin is a "mistake," arising out of ignorance of God's laws, then (c) reformation,

18. Joshua Jebb (1793–1863) was the British Surveyor-General of Prisons, well known for his design of the "model prison" at Pentonville, which opened in 1842 and set the standard for future prison construction. He was a friend of Nightingale's family; she consulted with him and incorporated some of his ideas in her *Notes on Matters Affecting the Health, Efficiency, and Hospital Administration of the British Army* (1858).

19. A member of Parliament for many years, Anthony Ashley Cooper, Earl of Shaftesbury (1801–1885) was one of the greatest philanthropists and social reformers of the Victorian age. An ardent supporter of sanitation, he wrote the instructions for the Sanitary Commission which the government sent to the Crimea in February 1855 at Nightingale's request.

20. Ragged Schools, established during the early to mid-nineteenth century under religious auspices, provided basic education and trade skills for poor and neglected children. They represented an attempt to integrate into society those who might otherwise resort to crime. In 1846, Lord Shaftesbury took on the presidency of a coalition, the Ragged Schools Union, which he vigorously promoted until his death. Nightingale was one of the supporters of the Ragged School at Westminster (BM Add. MSS. 45794.f65); the pupils printed a pamphlet she wrote about Kaiserswerth in 1851.

not punishment, is the only response to criminal behavior which is consistent with God's plan for humanity.

In Nightingale's view, the criminal is a "pioneer" in the sense that he or she charts unknown territory by demonstrating the undesirable consequences of certain actions:

> The pioneer's is the highest calling, and God calls the highest men to it. But the thieves and murderers who are also His calling, who are in some sense, His pioneers! how much more difficult it is to understand that He can have called them to such far greater agonies! It is probably this which has given birth to the expression that He Himself descends into hell with them. He could not call them to go alone. St. Vincent de Paul seems to have had an inkling of this truth, when he summoned his missionaries to the galleys "to visit the Son of God suffering for our crimes, in the person of these men who suffer for their own disorderly life.[21]

Nightingale comments below on the hypocritical attitude in Victorian England toward prostitution. She had come into close contact with prostitution around the hospitals and soldiers' barracks during the Crimean War and, according to Woodham-Smith, "the quality of her mind, her common sense, her humanity freed her from contemporary prejudice."[22]

At the time of the publication of *Suggestions for Thought*, prostitution was widespread and there was general disagreement about how "fallen women" should be treated. Some thought that prostitutes were sinners and criminals and should be punished accordingly. Others, like Nightingale, thought that prostitution was a product of circumstances and that it would decline if the social situation were changed so that more opportunities were given to women. In addition, by improving the plight of soldiers, morals would be raised and prostitution would decline. Still others felt that prostitution was inevitable and should be regulated so as to prevent the spread of syphilis and other venereal diseases. Those holding the latter opinion, which included the officers in the Army Medical Department, supported the Contagious Diseases Act (modeled on the continental system), which would require prostitutes to be licensed, forced to submit to medical examination on demand, and detained in hospitals for treatment. Nightingale was famil-

---

21. *Suggestions for Thought*, vol. 3, p. 71. Vincent de Paul (1581–1660) was founder of the Vincentian (or Lazarist) Congregation and of the Daughters of Charity. As chaplain of the French galleys, he worked to alleviate the suffering of the galley slaves.
22. Woodham-Smith, *Florence Nightingale*, p. 267.

iar with this system and considered it immoral and unworkable. She therefore used all her influence, both in government and military circles, to defeat the passage of the act in Parliament. She failed, however, and the Contagious Diseases Act became law in 1864. Social reformer Josephine Butler (1828–1906) took up the campaign against the act until it was finally repealed in 1886.[23]

At the end of this section, Nightingale comments on the lack of opportunity for any woman to develop her potential in the world. The concept of "spiritual starvation," introduced here, is poignantly developed in Chapter 5, "On Family Life."

∗　∗　∗

What has "society" done for us? What is the mission of society? of mankind? to civilize and educate us. How does it fulfil this mission? What does it do for "fallen women?" Those who have committed indictable crime, it takes possession of, and ordinarily condemns to a place where they must lose all hope as well as all desire of reformation. One would have thought that society, which had done so badly for them in their childhood, would now have wished to re-model them. Not at all. That is not the question. To punish them is all that is wanted. They must go, where the poisoner becomes corrupted and the forger loses all feeling, divine and human. They must be punished by being deprived of all lingering claims, to being thought human creatures and our sisters. "From him that hath little shall be taken away even that which he hath." But if indictable crime has *not* been committed, what does society do? What protection does she give those wretched women? What constraint does she put upon those men who make them what they are? Does she even turn a shy look upon them? Not at all. On the contrary, she throws open her doors wide to them, vicious as they are, and like the beggars, whom she puts in prison, while she praises those who give to them (curious anomaly!), so she says to the woman, "Get out of my path." While to him without whom the woman would not have been vicious, she offers her drawing-rooms and her high-bred daughters. Society takes pleasure in stimulating passion in every kind of way, by early excess in wine, late hours, school-boy conversation and classical books, &c. &c., and then says, "you must not gratify this in a

23. Paul McHugh, *Prostitution and Victorian Social Reform*; Judith R. Walkowitz, *Prostitution and Victorian Society: Women, Class and the State.*

legitimate way, under pain of exciting our censure—the illegitimate satisfaction is the only one we allow." And then she gives these satisfactions,
"like lilies, with full hands"—and allows no difficulty to remain unre-
moved.

But, if a criminal is great, if, by some political trade, he has, like
Schwarzenberg,[24] made himself useful to the designs of a government, of a
sovereign, then he does not go to prison or to Norfolk Island at all; on the
contrary, the "Times" writes of him that he will be remembered with
gratitude, if not with love. Society punishes a Rush and protects a Schwarzenberg.[25]

And we who are not "fallen women," we talk about mankind creating
mankind,—what has mankind done for us? It has created wants which not
only it does not afford us the opportunity of satisfying, but which it
compels us to disguise and deny. It affords us neither interest, nor affections, nor employment. Society neither finds us with work, if we are too
weak to find it for ourselves, nor with training to perform it, if we have
found it nor does it so much as suffer us to follow a vocation of our own,
not even if there be one too strong within us to perish for lack of nourishment.

It has made rich and poor, without teaching the rich to use their riches,
nor the poor their poverty. It says, if any one dies of hunger, "you must not
starve—so and so shall be punished if you do;" or "you shall be provided
for at the expense of society." But it never says, "you shall not starve
spiritually—you must not want the bread *of life*—so and so shall be punished if you do, if you lack the satisfactions which are as necessary to the
faculties and feelings as food is to the physical wants."

V

If the existence of universal law be granted, then *remorse* is not a true
feeling—not a feeling of what really *is*; for remorse is blame to ourselves for
the past. But if the origin of our will, and our will itself, were, as it has been
in accordance with law, there cannot, in truth, be blame to ourselves,
personally, individually.

24. Felix Schwarzenberg (1800–1852), Austrian prime minister, fostered the development of absolutism in the Hapsburg Empire by dissolving the Reichstag and abolishing the
constitution.
25. James Blomfield Rush (d. 1849), a tenant farmer, murdered Isaac Jermy (1798–1848),
the owner of the estate on which he worked, and Jermy's son. Evidently, Nightingale is saying
that Schwarzenberg's political intrigues make him as much a criminal as was Rush.

A distinction should be made as clearly as possible between absence of blame in an individual to himself, where he is conscious that he has been wrong, and indifference to that wrong.

To a healthy moral nature, having on an occasion erred, it would be as impossible to be indifferent to that error, though he should believe that it had not been in his possibility to avoid it, as it would be to one who should receive a bodily wound to be indifferent because it was not his fault.

We object to saying that a man *could* not have willed otherwise than he did, because this sounds as if he would or might have willed otherwise, but was under a necessity imposed by other and external power. We mean that the conditions on which will depends were such that, law being what it is, it was not possible that other will than that which did exist should exist.

We are most anxious to show that such an understanding of law, as manifested in human will and act, does not lead to indifference to right or wrong, but the contrary.

For a man to give way to feelings of remorse—of blame for what it has not been in him to prevent—is *not* true. To be conscious that wrong is wrong—to hold it in repugnance as all that we have to fear or avoid in our life and being—*is* true.

The more our state of being is human, manly, in the proper sense of those words,[26] the greater will be our repugnance to what is morally wrong, till wilfully to do wrong shall become an impossibility. The mind will *accord* with right, which is God's thought or consciousness, or will thirst and long and strive to do so, not in fear of His anger, but in love of right—of God, the living consciousness of right. Indifference to wrong is in the moral nature as blindness, paralysis in the physical nature, and would not follow as the consequence of believing that right is our health and weal; that it is conditional—that, if ignorant—if unable, either from want of will, of knowledge, or of power, to keep those conditions—we fall into our greatest, our only essential harm. Such a belief would lead to the pursuit of right, as including all man has to desire; to avoidance of wrong, as including all man has to avoid.

Our experience is, that to dwell on the past error with feelings of remorse depresses the energy, all of which is wanted to pursue the right in future.

When we are conscious of past mistake, whether it arose from ignorance of the right, or whether we had knowledge which might have di-

---

26. Nightingale is referring to the Sanskrit root word *manas*, "to think." Mankind is thus the "thinker," capable of understanding the universe and our place within it.

rected us, but had not will, let us set ourselves at once with all vigour to the life, the work of the present. Let us look upon the past as not almost but altogether springing from the righteous law of God. Let us accept the suffering of our mistake, accept our present work. Let trust in the redeeming power of God's law to invigorate us. Let us not spare ourselves the full consciousness of our mistake, let us look at our error as far as it may help us to truth. Let us strengthen our consciousness that there is no good but in the true and the right. Let us work on, even through our own faults and mistakes, with a noble striving for accordance with God's universal work.

Away with regrets which have no true foundation, empty your heart of them! Work out the page of to-day with goodwill, even though the mistake of yesterday may have complicated it. That very mistake shall lead to a brighter page than could have been, but that God, while his everlasting law of right secures us from all lasting evil, and assures us of all lasting good, gives to *us* to work the divine out of the human, to transmute ignorance into knowledge and feeling of truth.

But shall we have motive to avoid error, if we cease to suffer the pangs of regret and remorse?

There is a higher, better, truer help than those pangs—you will never rise high goaded by them. Strive to awaken the divine spirit of love in yourself, to awaken it in doing your present work, however you may have erred in the past—this will help you far better than dwelling on your own mistakes. There is nothing elevating or animating in the dissection of *them*. Essentially, in their very nature, they bring suffering or privation. Bear it in a true spirit, and work on. Turn your mistakes to as much account as you can, for the gaining of experience, but, above all, work on, yield not to paralyzing, depressing retrospection. God gives us the noble privilege of working out His work. He does not work for us. He gives us the means to find the way we should go. An eternal course is before us.

Better indeed to suffer the pangs of regret than to be indifferent; but, in proportion as we are conscious that we are throwing our earnestness into the present, we may dismiss regret for past mistakes. In proportion as we are striving for the path of righteousness, we may cease to look back on our false steps, except for experience to avoid them in future. And, even for that purpose, we must be careful not to weaken ourselves by feelings of despondence and depression, and regret, when intending only to learn experience. Much of the power for work will depend on the mood in which we work. We must consult nature and experience as to how best we can animate and elevate the spirit in which we live. We shall seldom find the spirit for doing our best in the present by dissecting our past mistakes.

5. On Family Life

We want to give that which the family *promises* to give and does not. We want to extend the family, not annihilate it.

I

> From Nightingale's point of view, society should be in harmony with the essence of religion, which is "the tie, the binding, or connexion between the Perfect and the imperfect, the eternal and the temporal, the infinite and the finite, the universal and the individual."[1] Society should be organized in a way that would strengthen this tie, to allow the divine nature, inherent in all human beings, to emerge and flower. She was highly critical of conventional British society, especially the family structure, which she considered a "prison," and the Church of England which she felt neglected women. Instead of nourishing the God-like qualities within young people, she wrote, these institutions starved them to death.

*   *   *

Society triumphs over many. They wish to regenerate the world with their institutions, with their moral philosophy, with their love. Then they sink to living from breakfast till dinner, from dinner till tea, with a little worsted work, and to looking forward to nothing but bed.

When shall we see a life full of steady enthusiasm, walking straight to its aim, flying home, as that bird is now, against the wind—with the calmness and the confidence of one who knows the laws of God and can apply them?

What *do* we see? We see great and fine organizations deteriorating. We see girls and boys of seventeen, before whose noble ambitions, heroic

1. *Suggestions for Thought*, vol. 2, p. 181.

dreams, and rich endowments we bow our heads, as before *God incarnate in the flesh*. But, ere they are thirty, they are withered, paralysed, extinguished. "We have forgotten our visions," they say themselves.

But is it extraordinary that it should be so? For do we ever *utilize* this heroism? Look how it lives upon itself and perishes for lack of food. We do not know what to do with it. We had rather that it should not be there. Often we laugh at it. Always we find it troublesome.

To have no food for our heads, no food for our hearts, no food for our activity, is that nothing? If we have no food for the body, how we do cry out, how all the world hears of it, how all the newspapers talk of it, with a paragraph headed in great capital letters, DEATH FROM STARVA-TION! But suppose one were to put a paragraph in the "Times," *Death of Thought from Starvation*, or *Death of Moral Activity from Starvation*, how people would stare, how they would laugh and wonder!

II

In Victorian England there were two proper choices open to a young upper class woman: to stay at home and be subject to the will of her parents until they died, or to marry and have her inheritance pass into her husband's name. For Nightingale, both options were unsatisfactory. She could find no fulfillment at home, where her family (particularly her mother and sister for whom social success was the primary goal in life) had for years thwarted her attempts to study nursing. The other option, to leave the family by marrying, was certainly a possibility for Night-ingale. She had several serious suitors, among them Richard Monckton Milnes (later Lord Houghton), who her mother thought would be a perfect match. Florence herself loved him, but after a nine-year court-ship she refused his offer of marriage. In private notes she analyzed her reasons:

I have an intellectual nature which requires satisfaction and that would find it in him. I have a passionate nature which requires satisfaction and that would find it in him. I have a moral, an active, nature which requires satisfaction and that would not find it in his life. . . .

I know I could not bear his life, that to be nailed to a continuation, an exaggeration of my present life without hope of another would be intolerable to me—that voluntarily to put it out of my power ever to be able to seize the chance of forming for myself a true and rich life would seem to me like suicide.[2]

    The conflict between fulfilling herself and fulfilling the expectations of her family members was particularly great for Nightingale, who sincerely loved them and was sensitive to their needs. She was plagued by guilt and in a letter to her father she asked forgiveness of all she had "pained."[3] Unfortunately, the conflict was never fully resolved; it set the stage for her illness, which is discussed in a subsequent section.

    ✳   ✳   ✳

    The family uses people, *not* for what they are, nor for what they are intended to be, but for what it wants them for—for its own uses. It thinks of them not as what God has made them, but as the something which *it* has arranged that they shall be. If it wants some one to sit in the drawing-room, *that* some one is to be supplied by the family, though that member may be destined for science, or for education, or for active superintendence by God, *i.e.*, by the gifts within.

    This system dooms some minds to incurable infancy, others to silent misery.

    And family boasts that it has performed its mission well, in as far as it has enabled the individual to say, "I have *no* peculiar work, nothing but what the moment brings me, nothing that I cannot throw up at once at anybody's claim;" in as far, that is, as it has *destroyed* the individual life. And the individual thinks that a great victory has been accomplished, when, at last, she is able to say that she has "no personal desires or plans." What is this but throwing the gifts of God aside as worthless, and substituting for them those of the world?

    The prison which is called a family, will its rules ever be relaxed, its doors ever be opened? What is it, especially to the woman? The man may escape, and does. The cases where a child inherits its parents' tastes are so rare that it has passed almost into a proverb. The son of a celebrated man is never a celebrated man: the two Herschels,[4] the two Mills,[5] are mentioned

2. Quoted in Woodham-Smith, *Florence Nightingale, 1820–1910*, pp. 51–52.
3. *Calendar of Letters*, 2.A2,260.
4. The astronomers William Herschel (1738–1822) and his son John Frederick William Herschel (1792–1871). William's sister Caroline Lucretia Herschel (1750–1848) was a distinguished astronomer in her own right.
5. John Stuart Mill and his father James Mill (1773–1836).

as memorable exceptions. A son scarcely ever adopts his father's profession, except when compelled, as in the case of caste; and in the countries where caste prevails, the race deteriorates. How often a parent is heard to say, "All that I have done will go to rack and ruin when I am gone. I have none to come after me who will keep it up!" It is said that the chances are 200 to 1, where a man's immediate descendants consist of three children and three grandchildren, against there being found one among these six who inherits his tastes and pursuits.

The law of God, it seems, is *against* repetition. Whatever the family, whatever the similarity of education, circumstances, &c., repetition is never seen. And is this extraordinary? In chemistry, the mixture of two substances constitutes an entirely new substance, of which neither the colour nor any of the properties can be predicated from a knowledge merely of the colour or any of the properties of the two original substances. So, in the family, though there can be traced, it is true, the family character, the family likeness, yet the children are all strikingly unlike each parent, strikingly unlike each other. Here the analogy with chemistry *appears* to cease, for the product of two chemical substances is always the same, under the same circumstances. But, such are the minute differences of circumstances which we never estimate, that the analogy may still remain; and, as it is said that there are no two leaves alike upon the same tree, so, and much more, there never were created two human beings alike. Now, what do we do with these *un*likenesses? The family strives to make them all do the same thing. If one of the family, as often happens, is superior to the rest, the rest, and especially the heads of the family, seem to want this one to be one with them, as we try to be one with God; he is to devote all his talent and genius to forward their ideas, not to have any new ones; to put their opinions, their thoughts, and feelings into a better dress, a more striking light, not to discover any new light; and, above all, he is not to find out any untruth in their ideas, or think he has any new truth, "for there is no such thing!"

To help others by *living*—by being *oneself*, is not this the true meaning of sympathy, the true benefit of companionship? But, in general, we have to live by *not* being ourselves. And what a fatiguing way of life it is! When we are not afraid of being ourselves, when we suit the people we are with, when what we say and feel does not shock them or annoy them or frighten them, life is easy, life is improving, we make progress. Now, *how* often does this happen in one's own family, where one can rarely speak without implying blame of something, without knocking against some one's preju- dices? And can it be otherwise when people are chained up together for life, so close in the same cage? It is often said that you are less known by your own family than by any one else. Is it wonderful? There is much of which you can never venture to speak. "The extraordinary reserve which he (or she) maintained with his (or her) own family" are words so common that every one has heard them, and yet they are always uttered as if it were a solitary, or, as it is put, an *extraordinary* fact. "He is so much more agreeable out of his own family," is another common remark. And how often you see "his" countenance fall when he is speaking to one of his own kin! As long as the iron chain is drawn tight round the family, fettering those together who are not joined to one another by any sympathy or common pursuit, it must be so. It is often disputed what kinds of character like society. It is probable that those like it who can say aloud the things which they would think to themselves, if they were alone. But how few can do this at home! There is no tyranny like that of the family, for it extends over the thoughts.

* * *

Nightingale managed to escape from the "prison" of family life in 1853, when her father agreed to give her a yearly stipend of five hundred pounds. As the new Superintendent of the Institution for the Care of Sick Gentlewomen in Distressed Circumstances, she chose to take up residence at the premises on Harley Street in London. Her act of leaving home unfortunately precipitated an explosion in the family circle: Fanny screamed and lamented; Parthenope had hysterics and fainted; W.E.N., unable to tolerate the situation, withdrew to the Athenaeum Club.

It was Nightingale's dream to participate in a spiritually oriented society or community, in which people of like mind could join together as an extended family. This would fulfill, she thought, the need for individual development as well as that for close ties of affection. Although she managed to spend some time at Kaiserswerth and on retreats at Catholic convents, she never realized this dream. After only a year at Harley Street she left for the Crimea; on her return she devoted herself to her work and adopted the lifestyle of an invalid and recluse.

* * *

Merely to protest against ordinary family life is of no use at all,—will only shock people: you must show a better life.

We would not destroy the family, but make it larger. We would not prevent people from having ties of blood, but we would secure all that the family promises, by enlarging it.

Monasteries, according to their original plan, were a much larger circle than the family. For there people did meet for a common object: those who had a vocation for work went into a house which supplied their kind of work—for contemplation, into a house of contemplation. Afterwards they degenerated into places of idleness and vice. But, in their original idea, they were places where people who liked to work for the same object, met to do so; and the enormous rate at which they multiplied showed how they responded to a want in human nature. Each was employed according to his or her vocation; there was work for all; but there is no such possibility in the family.

We want to give that which the family *promises* to give and does not. We want to extend the family, not annihilate it. We want "not to destroy, but to fulfil" the hopes it holds out—to supply the sympathy, the love, the fellow-feeling, the tenderness which it offers to supply and does not. Where is there such rudeness as in a family? Everywhere but in our own family our feelings are regarded. Now, we want to make a family where there shall be companionship in work, mutual attraction, love, and tenderness, we want to make *God's* family. We would not take away *any*thing, we would enlarge and multiply.

But where is there such absence of tenderness, such constant contention as in a family? and the oddest part of the thing is that everybody thinks it peculiar to themselves.

No, certainly, family does not answer its purpose,—(nor is it likely it should among five or six,) we want to make it do so.

The law of God seems to be to scatter; "go forth and conquer the earth and possess it," He says. Marriage does this, sons do this. The only exception to this rule seems to be the unmarried daughters. *They* must stay at home—because in a half savage state of society it is taken for granted that men have injurious feelings towards women, therefore women must remain at home till they are married for the sake of protection, or till society is in such a state that they do not want protection. The only exception to this rule is when they are obliged to earn their own livelihood; then, when they have something to do, they are allowed to go forth, that is supposed to be a protection.

But the Exodus should always follow the Genesis. Generated by the parents, they should, when they are supposed to be *re*-generated, go forth,—but unfortunately then comes the Leviticus, a number of rules and laws must be laid down, because they always misbehave when they have gone forth.

We don't wish to force them *out of* the family, we only wish them to be where all their faculties will be best exercised, *wherever that is*. Surely it cannot be denied that these two things are necessary, viz., that we should come into free communication with mankind, so as to give us room for our sympathies to find a response, *and* that we should have all our powers called into the highest exercise. If these two things were, there would be happiness, because then we could find work and sympathies for ourselves.

III

Nightingale writes that a young woman, just like a young man, should come into her inheritance at age twenty-one and thus be able to direct the course of her future. Unlike many reformers of her time, she was not convinced that getting the vote would improve conditions for either rich or poor women. Economic reform was, for her, the solution. In a letter to John Stuart Mill (August 11, 1867), in which she refused his request to play a prominent role in the newly formed National Society for Women's Suffrage, Nightingale wrote:

That women should have the suffrage, I think no one can be more deeply convinced than I. . . . But it will probably be years before you obtain the suffrage for women. And, in the mean time, are there not evils which press much more hardly on women than not having a vote? . . .

Could not the existing disabilities as to property and influence of women be swept away by the legislature as it stands at present?—and equal rights and equal responsibilities be given as they ought to be, to both men and women? I do not like to take up your time with giving instances, *redressible* by legislation, in which women, especially married poor women with children, are most hardly pressed upon now. I have been a matron on a large scale the greater part of my life, and no matron with the smallest care for her nurses can be unaware of what I mean e.g. till a married woman can possess property there can be no love and no justice.

Is it not possible that, if woman-suffrage is agitated as a means of removing these evils, the effect may be to prolong their existence? Is it not the case that at present there is no opposition between the two elements of the nation—but that, if both had equal political powers, there is a probability that the social reforms needed might become a matter of political partizanship—and so the weaker go to the wall? I do not know.[6]

Nightingale did not use her influence to promote legislation for women's rights, however, nor did she fully support the major feminist issues of her day, for example, the entry of women into the learned professions, such as medicine. Nightingale's overriding concerns were public health reform and the development of professional nursing, and she focused all her energy in these areas. So, although her work improved the lives of countless women, Nightingale did not play a central role in the feminist movement of Great Britain.[7]

*   *   *

What are we to do with girls? It is vaguely taken for granted by women that it is to be their first object to please and obey their parents till they are married. But the times are totally changed since those patriarchal days. Man (and woman too) has a soul to unfold, a part to play in God's great world.

Marriage is supposed to exercise a magical effect upon the judgment— for a married woman of eighteen has more independence, and is thought better able to act for herself than a single one of thirty-six. But it is not to be the first object for a man "born into the world," nor for a woman either, when he or she is of age, to please the parents. There is a higher object than this for the being which is to be one with God. It is true the child must obey and ought to obey implicitly. The question is, then, *when* the child becomes of age. If this were left to the parents' discretion, they would, perhaps, with the best and purest intentions, declare that their children were never of age. Parents seldom think that their children are grown up, and the children who have made most advance, and are before their generation, will always be those whom conscientious parents are most tempted to restrain as "geniuses unfit to judge for themselves in the common affairs of life," because, naturally enough, they cannot understand them. We see parents building up obstacles in the way of their children as zealously as if it were their sole vocation! It is almost invariable that, when one of a family is

6. Letter to J. S. Mill, 11 August 1867. BM Add MSS 45787.ff38–42. Quoted in Vicinus and Nergaard, *Ever Yours, Florence Nightingale*, pp. 287–288.

7. Nightingale's views on some feminist issues are discussed by Woodham-Smith, *Florence Nightingale, 1820–1910*, pp. 305–312.

decidedly in advance of all the others, he or she is tyrannized over by the rest, and declared "quite incapable of doing anything reasonable." A man runs away from this,—a woman cannot. The one who ought to be at the top of the ladder is always at the bottom. It is not only against those esteemed physically insane that commissions of lunacy are taken out. Others have been kept unjustly in confinement by their well-intentioned relations, as unfit to be trusted with liberty. In fact, in almost every family, one sees a keeper, or two or three keepers, and a lunatic. Happy for the poor lunatics, if there are two of them in one family! They may combine. Those natures which have the strongest affections, and therefore cannot bear not to please the others, not to be in the same key with the others, follow where they ought to lead. It must not be left to parents' discretion to declare, when a child is able to act for himself. The law has not left it at the discretion of parents and guardians to decide when a man becomes of age. If it had, he never would have become of age. It has fixed this age at twenty-one. It has not said twenty or twenty-five, but advisedly, taking into consideration the experience of mankind, it has fixed upon twenty-one. Guardians are not left to say *when* a young man shall come into the possession of his property. If they were, some, self-interested, would like to keep him out of it for their own sakes; others, well-intentioned and conscientious, would think he was still a child and not fit to manage it. But the law says *twenty-one.*

Who is to decide when a young woman shall come into possession of herself? Not the parents, certainly. A woman of twenty-one ought to consider herself of age, as regards her own conduct. It may be too early for some, too late for others. The real age of regeneration varies, when the child, generated by the parents at the age of o, is *re*generated by reason and education. But in spite of the mistakes which will follow, it would be better for children if they no longer considered themselves under tutelage after twenty-one.

The connexion between parents and children, in its present state of transition, is a miserable one; yet we would not have it back to its old state, if we could. In former days, children called their parents "Sir" and "Madam"; in the present days, they call them, at least one of them, "Governor" or "Relieving Officer;" in former times, they did not sit down in their parents' presence; in these, mothers wait upon their daughters, and are vexed at once that the daughters do not do it for themselves, and that they are not grateful to them for doing it. In the last century, proposals of marriage for the children were made to the parents; the parents accepted or refused, often without the knowledge, generally without the consent, of the children; in this, a man asks the woman herself, without the previous knowledge, and sometimes even in the absence, of the parents. In the last century, the relation was therefore a much more definite and easy one. Implicit obedience was exacted and given; submission, not love, was demanded; silence, not gratitude, expected. Then it might truly be said that the responsibility rested with the parents; for they undertook, and were understood to act, in the stead and without the cooperation of their children.

But now with whom rests the responsibility? The parents assume that they have it, but without any longer the rights to support it. Many a mother of this day would speak (if her feelings were put into words) thus:—"My mother did not think of what her daughter thought; her daughter had no business to think, *she* thought in her stead. I allow my daughter to think, but I expect that she shall always think like me. That is the least she can do, in common gratitude, in return for all that I have done for her. I don't desire her to obey—no such tyranny can exist in the nineteenth century; but she is always to act as I should do. I don't wish her to submit; but I wish her to be, what I wish to be with God, one with me. I don't command her to be silent, but I expect that her opinion shall always be the same as mine. I am excessively indulgent, that is, I take immense pains (*my* mother took no pains of the sort) to make her happy, in my way; to please her, according to my taste; to do what she *ought* to like, not what she does like; to arrange what *I* think is good for her, not what interests her—and she is not grateful." In these days, it can no longer be, "Do unto others as you would be done by," but "Do unto others as *they* would be done by." In the vagueness of all things which belongs to this transition-time, the relation between parents and children is as difficult to find as your way in a London fog. The parents take responsibilities which they cannot perform; the children feel that they are not performed. The parents feel that they are going through a great deal for their children; the children that gratitude is exacted from them for that which does not make them happy. Both sides suffer equally from disappointment, and both are alike to be pitied. The mothers are disappointed that they are not loved; the daughters that they feel no attraction towards the parents; for we can only love that which is loveable to us. An uncomfortable age! The last one was better. But no, it was not. We could not go back to that, if we would; and we would not, if we could. Still we know our daughters wish that they were married, as we did, in order that they may exercise at least some of their faculties and attractions. And no wonder; that is the reason why *we* married; and they will have to run the same chance with *their* children.

See what is expected of the poor unfortunate mother, that she should be able to respond to all the wants and tastes of all her daughters; the parts which twenty people could not play must all be acted by her; she must be a poet with one, a woman of business with another, an artist with a third, a thinker with a fourth, in order to develop the capabilities of each; and why? because they are shut up in a family, without free scope to find and exercise their natural inclinations and powers.

Yet daughters are now their mothers' slaves, just as much as before; they are considered their parents' property; they are to have no other pursuit, nor power, nor independent life, unless they marry; they are to be entirely dependent upon their parents—slaves in the family, from which marriage alone can emancipate them. Mothers acknowledge this, even while feeling that they are the daughters' slaves too.

What we have to do is so vague that we are obliged often to keep our responsibilities, while we have lost the privileges to which they appertained, and which alone could enable us to perform them.

IV

Creative work, writes Nightingale, requires the whole of one's time. "Everything that has ever been done at 'odd moments' had better never been done." Her comparison (see below) of the artist Murillo and "Mrs. A.," he who had the time to develop his talent and she who did not, is similar to Virginia Woolf's story about Shakespeare's sister in *A Room of One's Own*.[8] Woolf writes that "the birds that sang in the hedge were not more musical than she was. She had the quickest fancy, a gift like her brother's, for the tune of words. Like him, she had a taste for the theatre." While the young man achieved fulfillment, however, the girl had to remain at home where she had no opportunity to develop her creative talents. She eventually killed herself because, as Woolf notes,

it needs little skill in psychology to be sure that a highly gifted girl who had tried to use her gift for poetry would have been so thwarted and hindered by other people, so tortured and pulled asunder by her own contrary instincts, that she must have lost her health and sanity to a certainty.[9]

8. This passage is from "Cassandra," with which Woolf was familiar, so it is possible that Nightingale's words were her inspiration.
9. Woolf, *A Room of One's Own*, pp. 49, 51.

While Nightingale lived to a very old age, the conflict between pleasing those she loved and fulfilling her vocation took a tremendous toll on her health. The exact nature of her illness is still undetermined.[10] Sir George Pickering, in his study of creative individuals who suffered from ill health, identifies it as a "psychoneurosis." Discussing her condition during the years following the Crimean War when she was completing *Suggestions for Thought*, Pickering writes:

It would be hard to find a more classical case. Attacks of breathlessness, palpitation, giddiness, induced by unwanted events or events that cause apprehension, are typical and this is what Miss Nightingale displayed. Her illness prevented her from seeing unwanted visitors, and her mother and sister in particular, who would have wasted so much of her time. . . .

Her illness also solved other problems. As she had been ordered to remain lying down till her pulse settled, she was confined to her bedroom and the couch in her sitting-room. She could not go out and visit the people with whom she was working. They had to come to her. Moreover because it was now apparent that an unwelcome visitor would bring on an attack, all visits had to be by appointment and such was her delicate health that some could not be arranged at all. This enabled her to plan her time so that she could use it in the way she desired and in that way only. . . .

Her illness proved an invaluable ally in another and most important respect. Her life was thought to hang upon a thread, and she could hope to live only a few months at most. And so all her projects assumed an even greater urgency. She worked with great concentration and efficiency for some sixteen hours a day. She expected her colleagues and helpers to do likewise. And such was the magic of her legend and the power of her personality that they did.[11]

*   *   *

"For joy that a *man* is born into the world," Christ says. And that *is* a subject of joy. But a woman must be born into the *family*. If she were born into the *world*, it would be joy too. But what joy is there in her being born into the smallest of all possible spheres, which will exercise perhaps no single one of her faculties?

Every one will say this is preaching doctrine subversive of all morality. But what right have a man and woman to absorb all the powers of four or

10. For recent interpretations of her illness, see Marian J. Brook, "Some Thoughts and Reflections on the Life of Florence Nightingale from a Twentieth Century Perspective" and Shirley Veith, "The Recluse: A Retrospective Health History of Florence Nightingale," both in Vern Bullough et al., eds., *Florence Nightingale and Her Era: a Collection of New Scholarship*.
11. *Creative Malady*, pp. 166–167, 171–172.

five daughters? The right is all the other way. If I have brought them into the world, *they* have the right to expect that their powers shall be exercised, their lives made worth having, opportunity given them for developing all their faculties. I brought them into the world without consulting them; they had no choice in it, and I ought to have thought of this, whether I was able to give them all this, before I did so. "The mother that bore you" is often mentioned as such a subject of gratitude; as if life were such a boon that the mere circumstance of *my* having given *you* life entails slavery upon you. But whether it is a boon or not depends upon whether parents can make it so for children. "Bore you" to what? To take care of me? By the beautiful arrangement of Providence that the good of one shall tend to the good of all, and *vice versa,* that one cannot be injured without injuring the whole, the parents are injured as well as the children by this absorbing of their services.

And how often is there unsuitableness in the characters of the members of the same family. Look round among the families you know, and see how many you know in which they do not think there is something very peculiar in them. "We do not go on well, but," &c.; "I should not like it to be mentioned, but," &c.; "there is something *'very peculiar'* about that child," "such an unusual reserve," or, "I know there is a *'peculiar'* deficiency in myself." Do you know one family where the mother has what may truly be called a beautiful relation with the daughter? One which you would call a very happy family, except the "happy family" in the cage which travels about? "If I had but children like so and so," we hear constantly said in private, "but mine are so *'very peculiar.'*"

"Robbed and murdered" we read in the newspapers. The crime is horrible. But there are people being robbed and murdered continually before our eyes, and no man sees it. "Robbed" of all their time, if robbing means taking away that which you do not wish to part with, slowly "murdered" by their families. There is scarcely any one who cannot, in his own experience, remember some instance where some amiable person has been slowly put to death at home, aye, and at an estimable and virtuous home.

With regard to time, however, it is often said that if people made the most of their odd moments, they would have not much to complain of,— but they waste their spare quarters of an hour so grievously.

The maxim of doing things at "odd moments" is a most dangerous one. Would not a painter spoil his picture by working at it "at odd moments?" If it be a picture worth painting at all, and if he be a man of genius, he must have the whole of his picture in his head every time he touches it, and this requires great concentration, and this concentration cannot be obtained at "odd moments," and if he works without it he will spoil his work. Can we fancy Michael Angelo running up and putting on a touch to his Sistine ceiling at "odd moments?" If he did he would have to take it out again. But the value of fresco is that this cannot be done, and that is one reason probably why great masters preferred fresco, and said that oils were only fit "for children and dogs." The very gist of fresco painting is that it should be all painted in at once from one master idea, not niggled and dawdled at.

The Chancellor Oxenstiern[12] is recorded to have written a folio volume during the ten minutes his wife kept him waiting for dinner every day.

It was not worth his writing, then, nor our reading. Everything that has ever been done at "odd moments" had better never have been done; even a letter, written in a "spare quarter of an hour" had better not have been written. Can *any* work requiring thought be done at "odd times?" Perhaps the mere writing what has been carefully thought out in the watches of the night,—yet hardly even that, to any good.

Then are we to do nothing with our odd times? Are we to waste the spare moments which make up the greater portion of a woman's life? If you are to do *any*thing, you must do it then, is again said.

When people give this advice, it sounds as if they said, "Don't take any regular meals. But be very careful of your spare moments for eating. Be always ready to run into the kitchen and snatch a slice of bread and butter at odd times. But never sit down to your dinner, you can't, you know." We know what *can* be done at odd times, a little worsted work, acquiring a language, copying something, putting the room to rights, mending a hole in your glove. What else is there? I don't know. Nothing requiring original thought: nothing, it is evident, which requires a form, a completeness, a beginning and an end, a whole, which cannot be left off "at any time" without injury to it, which is not "mere copying," in short.

When Beethoven wrote a bar, he must have had the phrase, the movement, the quick time which was to succeed, the slow movement which came before—the whole piece, in short, in his thought. And could he write a bar now, a bar then, at an "odd moment?" This is what we call being a "dilettante," when a man does work in that way, and most of the

12. Axel Oxenstierna (1583–1654), Chancellor of Sweden (1612–1654), was noted for his administrative reforms and diplomacy during the Thirty Years War.

works of Dilettanti had better not have been. Women are at most always dilettanti, and have women ever produced any original work, any, with a *very* few exceptions, which the world would not be as well without?

Many, indeed, are the stories told of great men mastering a whole science in their spare moments.

There are, no doubt, some minds which can work, and some employments which can be taken up at odd times—where it is *acquiring* which is to be done. But if there is no digesting done, or if there is no time for digesting afterwards, the acquiring perhaps is not of much benefit. or a mind may become so possessed with a subject that it can work at it at *all* moments, but then the moments cease to be "odd." The greater genius which cannot and ought not to work without seeing the whole of its subject before its eyes, the most important subjects of thought which require this, these cannot be referred to "odd moments." People get out of the difficulty by not having *any* subjects of thought, which require to be pursued at other than "odd times."

How, in a family, where the one has to wait for the other—where, if they have any amiability, the employments of every one are constantly called upon to give way—how can the members, excepting those who have professions, ever have anything but "spare moments?"

How indeed? We constantly hear it said, "So and so has given up all her music since she married, or her drawing,—what a pity, such a first-rate artist as she was!" A married woman cannot follow up anything which requires exercise, and if, even for such second-rate things as these, people cannot command the time necessary, how will they do for subjects of *thought*? And we are slower still to apprehend that we must rob you of the state of mind *with* which to think, than of the time *in* which to think. If visitors come in, the lady of the house often complains that she will not have time to do this or that, she does not complain that she will not be in a state of mind when they go, to do it, if it is something important and requiring thought. She settles *that* by not having anything important to think about.

Half the people in the world have, indeed, no power of thinking. "What does it matter to give me time for that which I cannot do?" is often said.

But "half the world cannot think," *because* they have never tried. How is it possible? People get up in the morning and come down to breakfast, can they think then? After that, they read the newspapers or write letters, or sit in a room reading a book, where everybody is reading bits out of their own book aloud, or talking, till luncheon. Then they ride or drive, then they read a book or write letters till dinner. Then they spend the evening together till bed-time. This is interspersed, for women, with housekeeping, and visiting the poor people; for men, the House of Commons, managing their estates, the bench, and the board. Now, how are you to think? When are you to think? Not sitting with your feet on the fender, that is only dreaming. Few, except Descartes, ever thought without a pen in their hands.

A mother will say to her daughter, "Now, my dear, all the people are gone, you have all the afternoon to yourself, you can go up and employ yourself in your own room." But is she in a state to think? Is not her power of attention all frittered away? If she has breakfasted in a crowd, if she has been standing about for two or three hours afterwards, not knowing whether she might go away or not, how is her mind in any condition to think after that time? Sir Walter Scott even did not write his novels in that way.

But we are not all Sir Walter Scotts, nor Michael Angelos, nor Beethovens. On the contrary, such geniuses only come once in a thousand years.

How do we know that? We are often struck by the richness of organizations at 17 or 18, and how they go off afterwards. We are oftener surprised by the power than by the poverty of young characters. In many families there is one with a great dramatic talent, another with a genius for music, and a third with one equally remarkable for the pencil; a fourth writes like Coleridge. Yet we know perfectly well that these will be neither Michael Angelos, nor Beethovens, nor Mrs. Siddonses,[13] nor Miltons. Why? Mrs. A. has the imagination, the poetry of a Murillo,[14] and has sufficient power of execution to show that she might have had a great deal more. Why is she not a Murillo? From a material difficulty, not a mental one. If she has a knife and fork in her hands during three hours of the day, she cannot have a pencil or brush. Dinner is the great sacred ceremony of this day, the great sacrament. To be absent from dinner is equivalent to being ill. Nothing else will excuse us from it. Bodily incapacity is the only apology valid.

A lady friend of mine and Michael Angelo both had a turn for architecture. Michael Angelo studied it. My friend never did. All she did was pure genius. To compare her with Michael Angelo, of course, does not come into our head for a moment. How could she be compared, indeed? The one

---

13. Sarah Kemble Siddons (1755–1831), English actress.
14. Bartolomé Estéban Murillo (161?-1682), Spanish religious artist.

had no possibility given her, the other had. But people never think of this. They think nothing of being in a *state of mind* to think a great thought, to do a great work. They will fritter away all their power; and then think they have enough to do anything *they* want to do with it. They will let others play with them all the morning, and then think, "I shall have the afternoon to myself." You may do your accounts, or you may play with the children, or you may read an idle book, but do anything important which requires thought you cannot. And therefore the best way is to give up all subjects of thought, and that is what people do.

V

It seems as if the female spirit of the world were mourning everlastingly over blessings, *not* lost, but which she has never had, and which, in her discouragement, she feels that she never will have, they are so far off.

The more complete a woman's organization, the more she will feel it, till at last there shall arise a woman, who will resume, in her own soul, all the sufferings of her race, and that woman will be the Saviour of her race.

Jesus Christ raised women above the conditions of mere slaves, mere ministers to the passions of the man, raised them by his sympathy, to be ministers of God. He gave them moral activity. But the Age, the World, Humanity, must give them the means to exercise this moral activity, must give them intellectual cultivation, spheres of action.

Was Christ called a complainer against the world? Yet all these great teachers and preachers must have had a most deep and ingrained sense, a continual gnawing feeling of the miseries and wrongs of the world. Otherwise they would not have been impelled to devote life and death to redress them. Christ, Socrates, Howard,[15] they must have had no ear for the joys, compared to that which they had for the sorrows of the world.

They acted, however, and we complain. The great reformers of the world turn into the great misanthropists, if circumstances or organisation do not permit them to act. Christ, if He had been a woman, might have been nothing but a great complainer. Peace be with the misanthropists! They have made a step in progress; the next will make them great philanthropists; they are divided but by a line.

15. Probably John Howard (1726–1790), English philanthropist and reformer in the fields of penology and public health.

The next Christ will perhaps be a female Christ. But do we see one woman who looks like a female Christ? or even like "the messenger before" her "face," to go before her and prepare the hearts and minds for her?

To this will be answered that half the inmates of Bedlam begin in this way, by fancying that they are "the Christ."

People talk about imitating Christ, and imitate Him in the little trifling formal things, such as washing the feet, saying his prayer, and so on; but if any one attempts the real imitation of Him, there are no bounds to the outcry with which the presumption of that person is condemned.

For instance, Christ was saying something to the people one day, which interested Him very much, and interested them very much; and Mary and his brothers came in the middle of it, and wanted to interrupt Him, and take Him home to dinner, very likely—(how natural that story is! does it not speak more home than any historic evidences of the Gospel's reality?), and He, instead of being angry with their interruption of Him in such an important work for some trifling thing, answers, "Who is my mother? and who are my brethren? Whosoever shall do the will of my Father which is in heaven, the same is my brother and sister and mother." But if we were to say that, we should be accused of "destroying the family tie," of "diminishing the obligation of the home duties."

He might as well say, "Heaven and earth shall pass away, but my words shall not pass away." His words will never pass away. If He had said, "Tell them that I am engaged at this moment in something very important; that the instruction of the multitude ought to go before any personal ties; that I will remember to come when I have done," no one would have been impressed by His words; but how striking is that, "Behold my mother and my brethren!"

*   *   *

Nightingale did not develop her idea of the woman who will be the "Saviour of her race" or her idea of the "female Christ." From her point of view, however, all great discoveries and achievements are the result of the Divine Spirit working within humanity. As human progress is a developmental process, the great works of particular individuals are not isolated events but are dependent on the "accumulated and accumulating experience of all mankind (see Chapter 1, "On the Concept of God," sections III and IV). If the female Christ were to appear, therefore, a change would have to occur in the circumstances and organization of the "female spirit of the world."

Virginia Woolf, in *A Room of One's Own*, wrote similarly that the common life is of the greatest importance:

For masterpieces are not single and solitary births; they are the outcome of many years of thinking in common, of thinking by the body of the people, so that the experience of the mass is behind the single voice.[16]

Thus "Shakespeare's sister" will only come when there is a change in the consciousness, that is, in the circumstances and organization, of women as a whole:

As for her coming without that preparation, without that effort on our part, without that determination that when she is born again she shall find it possible to live and write her poetry, that we cannot expect, for that would be impossible. But I maintain that she would come if we worked for her, and that so to work, even in poverty and obscurity, is worth while.[17]

16. *A Room of One's Own*, pp. 68–69.
17. *A Room of One's Own*, p. 118.

6. On the Spiritual Life

Unless you make a life which shall be the manifestation of your religion, it does not much signify what you believe.

I

Our religious creed consists in this—belief in an omnipotent eternal spirit of love, wisdom, righteousness, manifesting itself by calling into existence, by definite laws, beings capable of the happiness of love, wisdom, righteousness,—capable of advancing themselves and each other in divine nature—living in an universe in which, by definite law, the means and inducement are afforded which insure their advance through their own activity to humanity's blessedness.

Whatever contributes to the advance of man's nature from the imperfect towards the perfect, whatever helps ignorance to knowledge, helps us to know and feel the Father, to enrich His Holy Spirit as existing within each of us.

Is it not evident that it is the spirit of God within man which undergoes suffering and privation? For what do we know of the spirit of God but that it is a spirit of righteousness, wisdom, goodness, love, benevolence, as manifested in the laws of existence? and what is all suffering and privation but a counteraction of, a contradiction to, a limiting of these attributes?

Perhaps it may be susceptible of evidence that there is no existence which can be called human, in which these attributes do not exist. If we can trace as existing in man, limited only in degree, all that we know or can know of God, is it not evident that man is God "manifest in the flesh?" Perhaps, if man becomes wise enough, he may call out, by the organization of life and by education, whatever there may be of such attributes in every human being; and certainly it cannot now be denied that the *tendency* is to prove the existence of such attributes, wherever human nature exists.

Experience and consciousness teach us that that which comes to us through exercise of some part or parts of our nature is of more value than that of which we are passive recipients—or, rather, we may perhaps say that such is our nature that it is impossible for us to be passive recipients of any good thing. Should we not expect, then, that the will of God, or of goodness, for the beings whom His will calls into existence, would be a good original nature, well exercised in life? It may be shown that such is His will. Suppose we were to imagine that those beings, whom His will calls into existence, possessed the best of natures, viz., His own, and that God's laws were adapted to exercise these best of natures, as righteousness, benevolence, and wisdom decree. It is susceptible of evidence that such is actually the case.

Suppose the laws of the material nature discovered, suppose mankind, individually and collectively, through successive generations, earnestly seeking to keep them aright, can any one doubt that the limits, now existing to the exercise of the divine nature in man, would be enlarged? Is this fanciful? Does not experience warrant such a belief? Suppose that, instead of life being regulated ignorantly, with little definite purpose, mankind, individually and collectively, aimed to organize life so as to improve character, *i.e.*, so as to extend the limits of the divine in man: can we doubt that thus man would, by exercise for himself and his kind, become more and more divine?

Individual men are part of a whole, of mankind, of the Son. They are *attainers*, acquirers of what the Father is and has. They are in Him, one with him, in proportion as they attain to be and to know truth. Different parts of one whole are contributing to one purpose in the case of mankind. Mankind is transmuting itself into the divine by exercise through God's communication of the divine. Man is utterly incapable of anything, except in as far as he *receives*; but he can receive nothing except through exercise, *appropriate* exercise of his own nature.

*   *   *

Nightingale's conception of the spiritual life is based on the mystical teaching that "the imperfect is the Perfect limited by material relations or, in other words, that man is God, modified by physical law." This was not an abstraction for Nightingale but "the essence of common sense,"[1]

1. From the preface to *Notes from Devotional Authors of the Middle Ages*; quoted in Cook, *Life of Florence Nightingale*, vol. 2, p. 235.

grounded in the facts of experience. She observed that the human character changes through circumstances, and thus if the appropriate circumstances were created the God-like qualities latent in all human beings could be actualized. Although she offers some suggestions regarding the appropriate circumstances for realizing the Divine within the human, she states that they are not fully discovered because of lack of interest on the part of humanity.

Nightingale discusses the Sacrament of Communion—the partaking of the body and blood of Christ—in a metaphorical sense, Christ being the Universal Spirit of Goodness which the man Jesus embodied. Cook writes that of all church rituals, the Communion Service had the most significance for her:

> She had little interest in rites and ceremonies as such, and she interpreted the doctrines of Christianity in her own way; but she found great comfort in the Communion Service, as an expression of the individual believer's participation in the sufferings and the triumph of the greatest of the Mystics.[2]

During Nightingale's years as an invalid, Benjamin Jowett often traveled to London from Oxford to give her Communion. "I should like to give you the Sacrament whenever you would like to receive it," he wrote in a letter, "It is no fatigue & will do me good, I hope, as well as you."[3]

*   *   *

God communicates with us by His nature actually becoming ours. The Roman Catholic, who sincerely believes that he eats the body and drinks the blood of Him in whom God manifested himself—oh! well may he feel himself invigorated, ennobled, penetrated! What grand ideas; grand, because true, are these of the Divine manifested in the human—of the Divine received into, becoming part of, the human! In these working days for money, for the external, for the intellectual, exclusive of the spiritual, (we speak of the general, the prevailing spirit,) such ideas become forms, and when such are ridiculous. But how penetrated must those have been who first, genuinely, had the conception, who felt, who thought, whose imaginations helped them to conceive, that the Divine verily manifests itself in

---

2. Cook, *Life of Florence Nightingale*, vol. 2, p. 243.
3. 20 November 1887; quoted in Quinn and Prest, *Dear Miss Nightingale*, p. 306.

the human, partakes itself, becomes one with the human, descends into the hell of sin and suffering with and for the human, banishes sin and suffering by being "verily and indeed taken and received" by the human.

But this is all mysticism, it will be said.

Is it not fact, revealed by experience and no mysticism, that, if man takes the appropriate means, wisdom, goodness, benevolence, love, righteousness, become himself: those very attributes, the very same which he recognizes in God's laws, in the manifestations of God, in the communications with God? The spiritual and sincere Roman Catholic *did* receive these attributes, in receiving, as he supposed, the "body and blood" of the manifestation of the Perfect, for he raised his nature to think, not of the body and blood, but of the spirit. Let us try to enlarge and purify our conception, to remember our privilege of being invited *always* to this sacrament, to partake, to receive, to become one with the Perfect. Is it possible to deny that we have this invitation? He is ready to manifest Himself in us, as He did in Christ, to make us also Saviours, to partake Himself with us. We may be one with Him and with each other.

Man has not apparently cared to find out how most to increase in love and wisdom; not cared at least sufficiently to make it a definite object, as he has in regard to physical strength. Or he has not discovered that there are definite means for acquiring spiritual nerve and sinew as well as bodily. But man has unlimited means for spiritual advance. The eternal source of truth, of goodness, and wisdom is ever ready to supply the faculties of mankind with means of increase, so that to-day may always be richer than yesterday, if these means are taken. The bold metaphor, "Feed on Christ," is correct, if by Christ is meant the spirit of truth, love, righteousness.

II

Spirituality, according to Nightingale, is evoked by the recognition of a "higher presence" beyond that of the human and material, and by partaking of its nature. She criticized traditional means believed to strengthen spirituality, particularly ascetic practices such as fasting and mortification of the flesh. Having worked among England's poor, and having witnessed the fatal shortage of supplies during her time in the Crimea, it comes as no surprise that she rejected spiritual practices which renounce basic material needs. Nightingale instead approached

the spiritual life as she did nursing and social reform: knowledge is
obtained through observation and experience.

*　*　*

What do we mean by spirituality?

Is it not *feeling*, as distinct both from intellect and from the affection of
one human being to another? We do not call love, admiration, reverence,
for a human being, spirituality, nor the trust which one human being has in
another. These we call humanizing influences; but feelings called forth by
the consciousness of a presence of higher nature than human, unconnected
with the material, these we call spiritual influences; and this we are conscious is the highest capability of our nature. Whenever we love, admire,
reverence, trust this higher presence—whenever we sympathize with, partake in the purpose, thought, feeling, of this highest presence—these are
our best moments.

Sympathy with man, interest in any right or innocent object, is not
excluded by this higher state, is never indeed perfectly right and healthy,
except in connexion with it.

There *are* modes (all in accordance with law) of vivifying and strength-
ening spirituality.

Fasting and prayer are usually supposed to be these modes. All undue
or inappropriate care for anything does indeed check spirituality. The saints
discovered this, experimentally, no doubt. So they took to banishing agreeable food and cheerful converse, even where not wrong. Except in a few
great instances (St. Bernard, St. Ignatius Loyola, St. Vincent of Paul, &c.)[4]
denying the flesh its due made it only cry out, instead of leaving the being
free for highest things. But the wish, the seeking for spirituality, which
inspired a few among the saints, was, perhaps, higher than anything now
existing.

Many went to convents and hermitages, hoping to win heaven or ward
off hell; many to be applauded or to gain in some way in this world; many
thinking to do God service, or give Him pleasure by sacrificing *themselves* or
worshipping *Him*. But there is evidence that a few sought a spiritual state of
being as their object, which no Church, scarcely any individual, seeks now.

4. Bernard of Clairvaux (1090?–1153), French Cistercian mystic and Doctor of the
Church, wrote a number of important treatises including *De Diligendo Deo*. Ignatius of Loyola
(1491–1556), Spanish spiritual director and founder of the Jesuit order, is best known for his
Spiritual Exercises. For Vincent de Paul, see Chapter 4, note 21.

Spiritualism is dormant, not dead, let us hope. How to revive it, to rekindle it into life, is the great question.

The spirit of our operatives is far from being spiritual. It is quite in an opposite direction. So are all the tendencies of the age. In a much more ignorant and savage age it does not appear to have been so. Man goes a weary course *away* from spirituality while learning the laws and capabilities of matter. Is not the time come when he may return to it, with reason and knowledge as a foundation for what was before unconscious impulse?

It seems very strange that, when such men as St. Ignatius Loyola, St. Bernard, and Wesley, could find no peace without finding God, and travelled up and down the earth in search of Him; very strange that there should be some now denying that there is a God; others saying that *we* cannot know anything of Him, if he exists. A large majority of our world, at least in England, is very near losing His name. In the minority we hear much of the Name, but how often it is but a name, without any conception, or any attempt at conception, of the *character* of God. We accept what men called God long ago. We do not care to inquire whether the human mind, through its progress in different directions, might not receive enlightenment concerning God beyond that of past ages. "To proclaim the name of the Lord" was once felt a high mission. That name should now tell us of ONE more great and good than was then proclaimed. "Who shall by searching find out God?" There is true feeling in those words, if we accept them as indicating that we cannot find him out "to perfection." But there is great danger in them if they satisfy us in not seeking what *more and more* we may know and feel of God if we will.

To proclaim the *character* of the Lord, how he reveals it to us if we will—what a mission that would be for a Saviour of this day! The most moral and the most intellectual of the English artizans are now learning to live satisfied without Him, and really seem to think it does not signify His not being there. And they are not likely to feel any *want*. They live in a state of triumph. And they *have* morality; they have sympathy; they have benevolence; they will not feel these wants. If a man were alone, he might come to feel the want of God. But these say, "I don't know whether there is a God or not; but if there is, I cannot understand Him, and it is, therefore, no use to seek Him." It seems curious that it should be so, while others in former times have felt His presence—felt that it was the one essential to make life worth having, and that all else might be dispensed with if that remained. Oh! how to keep that sunshine in our hearts? Experience must show to each.

III

Nightingale returns to the idea that she put forth previously, that the human will is lawfully determined by the character and the circumstances of the individual. The development of spirituality, that is, the realization of the Divine presence, thus requires the keeping of certain conditions, not simply "willing" to be spiritual. She discusses various means for "growth in grace," such as the keeping of the Sabbath, common worship, the study of the Bible, and prayer.

For periods after Nightingale's youth, very little material is available on her personal participation in church services. After her return from the Crimea she avoided all public functions, including those of the church, but the humorous observations included below indicate that as a young girl she did, indeed, go to church. Nightingale had great respect for the Bible, even though she felt it contained errors (see Chapter 1) and could not be regarded as containing the ultimate truth. She spent a great deal of time helping Benjamin Jowett organize *The School and Children's Bible*, which was published in 1873,[5] and at the Nightingale Training School she had classes established for the study of the Scriptures. In Plato, however, she found a prayer which she found consistent with her philosophy and which she thought was unequaled by any Collect in the service-book. She wrote to Jowett that at least half the mystical teachings of St. John of the Cross, were contained in the short closing prayer of the *Phaedrus*: "Give me beauty in the inward soul, and may the outward and inward man be at one."[6]

*   *   *

Of all the fatal mistakes that have been made to impede the progress of the human race, this perhaps has been the most fatal, viz., the superstition that we have nothing to do but to exert the will, as it is called, and all former error will be rectified, all future good secured. If this mistake had been made with regard to the physical health, mankind would probably have come to an end. If we believed that a man with one diseased lung has nothing to do but to will, in order to have two good ones; if we believed

5. Quinn and Prest, *Dear Miss Nightingale*, p. 226; Cook, *Life of Florence Nightingale*, vol. 2, p. 228.
   6. Cited in Cook, *Life of Florence Nightingale*, vol. 2, p. 232.

that a man when he is hungry has nothing to do but to will in order to eat, the human race would soon perish. Are not the laws of the spiritual world at least as numerous, important, and worthy of study as those of the physical?

Take the common course of a drunkard. He may abstain once, by force of conscience or even feeling, or some other motive, but his physical state, which has been accustomed to stimulus, will want it more at the end of 24 hours than of 12. We must consider the whole of the nature on which we wish to work, whether it be our own or any one else's. It is not enough to address yourself to the conscience, while, perhaps, the nerves, the spirits, which have also their laws, may be in a state of severe suffering, from want of the stimulus to which they have been accustomed. But what do we do? Twice a week, we say, we have done nothing we ought to have done, and we have done everything we ought not to have done (in order to make sure of leaving nothing out). And we mean, to lead an entirely new life from this moment, to do something entirely different. But it is very certain that we do not, because we intend to say the same thing again in the afternoon. The science of moral recovery is at least as intricate as that of physical recovery.

To think that we can be good under *any* circumstances is like thinking that we may be healthy when we are living over a sewer. If a person has to go to an unhealthy climate, he does not say, "I can be well if I choose under any climate," but he takes means, as far as he can, to arrange other healthy circumstances. If the heat is intense, he takes care to have exercise in the early morning; if the dews are hurtful, he takes care not to be out just at sunset; so there may be circumstances under which a man cannot be good and yet which he cannot, at present, rightly alter. In that case it is not by saying, "I can be good, if I only will, under any circumstances," that he will maintain himself so; but by supplying, as much as in him lies, circumstances which will make him so.

Here, again, comes in that fatal mistake about the will. The boy William is good and happy in some occupation for which he has a vocation, that is, to which God calls him. If it is right for the convenience of parents or for the conventional code that he should adopt some other occupation, parents seldom hesitate to say, "This is not the thing for you, go and be good and happy in the Law, or the Church, or at College;" and they would not doubt but that it was in his power to say, "I *will* go and be good and happy in the Law, or in the Church, or at College." To *say* it is, indeed, in his power, and, if he is amiable and feeling, he will probably try to say it; but to *be* it may not be in his power; and this is just the practical mistake which shows the want of a true conception about the will. It is taken for granted that there is this uncomprehended something, called will, which what we call William can command, what we call will will obey, without our understanding what man is, what the man William is, what the will is; and thus among well-intentioned people, half the mischief in life arises. What a dangerous immoral doctrine, people say, that we are in the hands of circumstances. No, we are in the hands of God.

"I can be good if I will," is the road to despair; for a person says, "I will be good when I go back to such and such circumstances; I resolve to be good; I know I can if I will." He "wearies Heaven with prayer;" he fails and fails; he thinks the fault lies in his will, and he sinks lower and lower till he gives himself up as lost.

But we don't *only* say "will!" There are "means appointed" for our "growth in grace."

Observance of the Sabbath

"To-morrow is Sunday!" and what a curious thought that to-morrow, in all the length and breadth of Christendom, people will put on their best clothes, and be in time for church, and think that they have performed a duty by going to church, and hardly anybody will really feel anything whatever, when there.

And what is the cause of its being Sunday to-morrow all over the Christian world? Why is Sunday kept?

From the feeling of a Superior Being.

But why does that make people put on their best clothes?

Out of a feeling of respect to Him.

But we appear to think this Superior Being more particular about the fashions than about the arts, for there is such singing in the church as you would not suffer for a moment in your drawing-room. Such reading aloud there is as you would not allow in your own family; nowhere is such reading as the clerk's ever heard, except in church. "Let us sing to the honour and glory of God," and then such music follows as is certainly not to the honour and glory of the singers. Then, although the people are dressed in their best, the church is not; it is generally so uncomfortable, ugly, and bare a place that you would not go into it, if it were not the house of God. God's house is much dirtier and shabbier than anybody else's house. We feel so strongly the necessity of a Sabbath—a day of rest—a day peculiarly devoted to religious thought and feeling and to their expression by God's children gathered together, that surely, whatever external aid is called in from art, as music, architecture, &c., should be of the best.

One day in seven set apart by common consent of all the world for finding out the spiritual laws of God is indeed an inestimable advantage. We should like to have two. Even in discovering the material laws which everybody acknowledges to be very important, how many hindrances people find, in consequence of the consent of mankind not being with them. Some are hindered by hunger, others by the "laws of conventional society," unfortunately not the same as those of God. Those who are prevented by the fear of starvation, and those who are frightened by that of being "thought odd," are therefore equally out of the pale of true discoverers. Now, a Sunday which is granted by universal consent both to the very poor and the very rich is inestimable. Only let us use it as such.

WORSHIP

As to a "common worship" as it is called, instead of having it once a week, we would have it every day, twice a day. The word "*worship*," however, seems hardly to express what God wants of us. He does not want to be praised, to be adored, to have his glory sung. We can scarcely conceive a good man, a very limited edition of God's perfections, wishing it. How inappropriate, then, to Him all this praise! And many only give it, because they are afraid of Him, for how can He be really thought good, with such qualities as are ascribed to Him, vanity, anger, revenge.

What he desires seems to be accordance with Him, that we should be one with Him, not prostrate before Him.

"Submitting to God's will" is a phrase we cannot understand. It is as if you looked upon God as something apart, *without*, independent of all principle, to whom you have only to submit. But if, for "God," we read "the spirit of perfect love and wisdom," how can we talk about *submitting* to perfect love, directed by wisdom? We accord with it; we don't submit. It is often said, "So-and-so is so good, she submits entirely to God" as a *merit*. In so far as she is good, she is part of the divine goodness, accordant with it, willing the same things, omnipotent in as far as she wills the same things. Is it not a mistake to call this submission? It is *oneness*. Christ's will was God's will—the will of love.

I would try to teach a child—not to "submit" to God, nor to pray that anything should be otherwise—but to second Him. I would try to inspire it with the idea that it, the child, can second GOD!

BIBLE

What is morality to be referred to? Is it not to our sense of right? But we have referred it to a book, which book makes many contradictory assertions. Discoveries are being made every day in physical science; but in the most important science of all no discoveries are made or can be made. Why? because the book is final. Supposing Moses had written a book about mechanics, and this book was regarded as the ultimatum, we should have made no progress in mechanics. Aristotle was supposed to have written such a book, and for 1,800 years people disbelieved their own actual experience before their eyes, because they could quote chapter and verse of Aristotle to a contrary effect. Yes, with the sound of two weights falling simultaneously in their ears, they maintained that the weight which was ten times heavier than the other fell in one-tenth of the time of the other, because *Aristotle had said so.* Is not this an exactly parallel case?

Religion under this view, it will be said, will consist partly of assertions considered to be proved, partly of subjects for further consideration among mankind. Much is to be learnt from the Bible, and probably from all books which have been accepted by large portions of mankind as inspired; but man's capabilities of observation, thought, and feeling exercised on the universe, past, present, and to come, are the source of religious knowledge.

PRAYER

It did strike me as odd, sometimes, that we should pray to be delivered "from plague, pestilence, and famine," when all the common sewers ran into the Thames, and fevers haunted undrained land, and the districts which cholera would visit could be pointed out. I thought that cholera came that we might remove these causes, not pray that God would remove the cholera.

I gave up praying, in the sense of *asking,* from experience, and not from theory.

Observing whether prayer was answered, and finding it was not, it occurred to me that this was not God's plan, that His scheme for us was not that He should give us what we asked for, but that mankind should obtain it for mankind; that we were not paupers asking at a Poor Law Board for relief, but men working for themselves and their fellow-creatures.

It will be said, if we are to have no prayer, we lose our chief support and comfort in this painful world.

But what is the intercourse we now have with God? Prayer, in its present sense, is to give utterance, at stated times, to a form of flattery and to selfish or unwise requests. It is, as in the Litany, to say to God, "Don't go this way, don't go that way," till we have marked out the whole line which He ought to go, and interdicted to Him the fulfilling of almost every law which He has made.

We want, it is said, the direct personal communication with God and Christ, that we may ask and hear them answer. Do not take from us, is the cry, our Saviour, the Christ who died upon the cross for us.

And does not God do much more than die upon the cross for us? Is He not in every one of us, going through sin and suffering, "descending into hell" with us? Does he not suffer, not once for us, but every day in us? And can we want anything more than communion with the perfect and eternal Father?

I want, it is said, communion with Christ, my divine brother, who feels for me.

And you will have it with the Son, the divine in man, with many Christs, who suffer for all mankind.

But we want a Son "to make intercession for us."

Do you suppose that Christ is ever "making intercession" for us? It is true He "ever liveth," to work for us, but—to "intercede" for us? He had better not exist at all, God had better not exist at all, than be employed in this way; the one in persuading, the other in being persuaded.

But we want an answer. It is no comfort to say that God may hear me, but He does not speak to me. Man wants an answer.

Can he receive it from the Eternal when he cannot comprehend what eternity is,—from the Infinite and Perfect, when infinity and perfection are beyond his understanding? Were God to speak to him, could he hear? Were God to tell him His plans, could he comprehend them?

But God does not refuse to answer the longing, devoted spirit, which says, Speak, Lord, for thy loving child heareth. He hears as the Father; He answers as the Son, and as the Holy Spirit. I could not understand God, if He were to speak to me. But the Holy Spirit, the Divine in me, tells me what I am to do. I am conscious of a voice that I can hear, telling me more truth and good than I *am*. As I rise to *be* more truly and more rightly, this voice is ever beyond and above me, calling to more and more good.

But you have to invent what it says.

We believe that each man has his Holy Ghost; that is, the best part of himself inspired by God. But whether it is I who speak, or whether it is God speaking to me, I do not know. We call upon our fellow-creatures to study this subject. That Prayer, as *asking*, will entirely cease, we are certain. If we give up *asking, confessing* our sins and formal *praising*, will it be said, what remains to be expressed to God? Surely, infinite are the sympathies, infinite the thoughts and feelings, of man towards the Perfect Spirit, with whom he desires to be one.

Let us think what we should ask God to communicate, if we believed He would hear us, and grant what we ask.

Of that which is asked every day much is impossibility, because to grant it would be a contradiction to truth and wisdom. Much that we ask we shall certainly receive, because it is accordant with truth and wisdom that we should receive it; but is *asking* the true intercourse to hold with the Perfect, who is always telling, always offering all things?

We will *ask*, then, nothing of God. How ungracious, how stupid it is to ask the Gracious, the rich Giver, the wise Father, who is always offering all. But we will seek continually (and stimulate mankind to seek with us) to prepare the eye and ear of the great human existence, that seeing it *shall* perceive, and hearing it *shall* understand. "Seek and ye shall find"—seek *wisely* must be added—"knock, and it shall be opened,"—knock, *i.e.*, not against a stone wall made to remain a wall, but at a door made to open.

It is development which we seek—development from the imperfect towards the perfect—from ignorance towards truth. And how is this to come? By the will of the All Wise it is to come by means, by the appropriate exercise of the nature. *Prayer* has sometimes been such exercise; it has been a wish after the right and good, a referring to God as the source of the true and good. We say, and say truly in this sense, what religion can exist without prayer? None can exist without reference to the Source of all for all—none without wish to partake what He is; and, in as far as prayer seeks Him and refers to Him, it is an essential of religion.

Ask of perfect wisdom, you will have an answer above and beyond yourself. Speak, articulately or inarticulately, to perfect goodness and love, such existence hears you, answers you, through the exercise of your own nature, it is true, but it is not your own nature which answers you, but a higher. It is not the mere fact of using words which brings this answer. Many, many are the words spoken to this Holy Spirit which receive no response. Time has already disclosed conditions which, if kept, allow a communication between the holy spirit of God and the holy spirit in man. It used to be thought that God spoke occasionally to individuals, with no other condition than that it was His arbitrary will so occasionally to speak—that He called man out of his sleep with no reference to any particular state in man, the consequence of which would be always communication of the divine in man with God.

But experience shows that there are times when man may ask this communication, but cannot have it, because the conditions for having it have not been kept. But let him have patience to find out and to keep these conditions, and wisdom, and love and goodness, which he will feel above his own, will dwell with him; he may interpret their words.

Evidence for this may be found in experience. We believe, from experience, that man is capable of living always, as it were, in a state of reference to that higher Being—that, as the world's ways improve, far as we are from it now, man's intercourse with man will be regulated so as to help this higher intercourse, to keep it unbroken, whereas now it is almost impossible not to break it as soon as man is with his kind.

Deep souls who wanted it fled to wildernesses, to monasteries, and as always happens, others who did not comprehend them, imitated them, and fleeing from the world became a fashion; although it is hard to understand what it means, since the world is what we have to mould, not to fly from.

It is said that mysticism is mistaken in urging man to isolate himself with God, and devote himself exclusively to his Creator; whereas man's natural inclination, implanted in him by God, urges him to devote himself to his fellow-man, urges all mankind mutually to unite in benevolent ties. But those who say this do not see that the first motive for mankind to unite is devotion to God; that devotion to God is the spring of love to man, makes it necessary, is the same thing. One with God, one with man.

*   *   *

As seen in the foregoing section, Nightingale consistently utilizes the terminology of the Christian Trinity (Father, Son, and Holy Ghost or Spirit) in her references to God. The Trinity was a concept which Nightingale had pondered on her trip to Egypt when she noted its presence in ancient thought. Comparing it to the Christian doctrine, she wrote:

We make a distinction almost similar between Father, Son, and Holy Spirit, when we call the Father the thought, the Son the word, and the Holy Ghost, if I may say so, the hand, i.e. the worker, the communicating medium. As, with us, the First Person of the trinity arranges, the Second commands, the Third actuates or vivifies.[7]

---

7. *Letters from Egypt* (1854 edition), pp. 86–87. (The 1854 edition contains many more references to the Trinity than does Sattin's edition.)

In *Suggestions for Thought*, however, she remarked that "the words 'Father,' 'Son,' and 'Holy Ghost,' are wearisome to many," and they are used "in a widely different sense from what we should wish to do." Rather than using "Father" to represent an anthropomorphic Godhead, she spoke of the Father as being wisdom, goodness, love, righteousness, and power. He is moreover the thought, purpose, and will that engenders *development*.

The Son, she indicated, is the manifestation of God, that is, humanity, which *develops* according to the will of the Father, such that the Son's nature actually becomes that of the Father. "The Father," she wrote, "is at all times making Himself the Son, God becoming man to enlighten us."

The "Holy Ghost," in her view, seems to denote something of the divine within each individual through which the Father communicates His will to the Son. "Let us distinguish," she wrote, "God the Father as the spirit of perfection, incomprehensible to us; God the Holy Ghost, as what is comprehensible to each man of the perfect spirit." She summarized the relationship between the three elements of the Trinity as follows:

. . . the Son must work his way from ignorance and imperfection to truth and perfection before he is one in being with the Father. The holy spirit developed within him by the law within and around him shall lead him onwards till his being is one with God. Then shall the spirit of God again set forth on the work of fresh development and manifestation.[8]

Although Nightingale clearly believed in the human existence of Jesus, at times she seems to have regarded Christ as the embodiment of a level of consciousness, declaring that Marcus Aurelius, Moses, and Christ are three words for the same thought,[9] as if this "spirit of truth, love and righteousness" manifested itself in these three individuals. While she rebuffed the traditional view of Christ as a divinely appointed "messenger," she did view him as the perfect prototype for mankind because "Christ's nature harmonized with God's nature." As seen in the following passage, she viewed Christ in both a spiritual and human light, and sternly criticized prevailing concepts of Christ.

8. *Suggestions for Thought*, vol. 1, p. 114.
9. *Calendar of Letters*, 2.C13,372.

But what a character his was! When he talks about the baptism and the fire he has to go through, how expressive those words are! A baptism of fire he might well have called it. Every person must be baptized with fire who would do anything which is not usually done in the conventional walk of his life, which is not provided for in the ordinary course of things. Every person must have a baptism of fire who is not satisfied with the world as it is, and who would fain help it out of its rut. "And how am I straitened till it be accomplished!"

But there are many things he said, which are very beautiful, and yet are not true. When they brought the woman taken in adultery before him, and he turned aside and wrote in an absent mood on the ground, and then said, "he that is without sin among you, let him first cast a stone at her"—that beautiful tender spirit felt truly. But still there is a right and a wrong about adultery. This would be putting an end to all law and justice. If no one is to execute the law unless he be perfectly pure himself, the Lord Chief Justice and the Chief Baron must vacate their seats on the bench, and the police be disbanded, and the criminal jurisprudence of a country come to an end.

And when he implied that we should take no more thought than the lilies of the field, is that absolute truth?

And what he tells the Samaritan woman of the "living water" is very beautiful, but when she does not understand, he seems to make no effort to explain to her. He was so filled and absorbed with his own thought that he seems to have spoken absently, and hardly to have cared whether she understood or not. He even sometimes says, "That seeing they may see, and not perceive, and hearing they may hear, and not understand." Might not the people have said, if you are to teach us, would it not be better to speak so that we can understand?

What a point he seems to have made about faith, believing that we can do a thing! "Faith can remove mountains." Now, it is very true that very often we do not believe we can do a thing, which, if we did believe it, we could do. But we may believe we can do a thing which we can't. A great many, from ignorance of the laws of God, have done so. Believing does not make us able to do it; does not make the law of God by which to do it. He seems to have known the first fact, and to have confused the second with it.

But what have we made of Christ in these vulgar times? We have daubed him all over with bright colours, so that we can hardly see through to the original beautiful form underneath. The churches have made him a God, and said, What! do you think you are like Christ? while they are preaching you to imitate him. The Unitarians have made him a perfect man, preaching that of which you see a great deal is not true. If we could but show him in his original form! The idea of a divine being dying to save you from another being does excite some feeling; but to tell you to listen to preaching which is perfect, and which you see is imperfect, and the whole of which you *cannot* believe, excites no feeling at all. If he is to be merely a teacher or merely a God, he is nothing.

IV

Humility and pride, Nightingale writes, are two extremes that should be transcended by an honest appraisal of one's abilities. Nightingale herself did not depreciate the value of her contribution during the Crimean War, but she did admit that there was another person who would have done better. In a letter to the Mother Superior of the Bermondsey Convent, who, with four of her nuns, had been one of Nightingale's mainstays, she wrote:

I do not presume to express praise or gratitude to you, Revd. Mother, because it would look as if I thought you had done the work not unto God but unto me. You were far above me in fitness for the General Superintendency, both in worldly talent of administration, and far more in the spiritual qualifications which God values in a Superior. My being placed over you in an unenviable reign in the East was my misfortune and not my fault.[10]

Finding work for which one is suited and doing it "unto God" is Nightingale's active mysticism. Then pride and humility (and, indeed, one's own personal self) are forgotten in the light of a larger interest.

*   *   *

The parish clerk who said, "You may pray for rain, but it's no use while the wind is in that quarter," spoke according to experience and observation. In the same way we may pray for self-forgetfulness, but "it's no use" while the wind is blowing from the quarter of luxury and idleness. We may pray for humility, but "it's no use" while there is no wind of sufficient strength to blow our thoughts away from ourselves.

How many have struggled against a sin of vanity, and prayed and

10. Letter dated 29 April 1856. Quoted in Cook, *Life of FLorence Nightingale*, vol. 1, pp. 299–300.

prayed, and gone through years of self-mortification, and self-inflicted tortures, and wondered why God was so far off, and whether "His arm was shortened that He could not save" and why He was so deaf that He would not hear, and have been brought to the very verge of despair; "the sorrows of death compassed me, and the pains of hell gat hold upon me;" whereas if they had lived a life which had afforded them one interest so strong as to make them forget themselves, they would have forgotten their own puny reputation from the mere force of another interest.

In the same way with pride. The desire to be something, to do something, is implanted in us. Everybody ought to command. No one's faculties are fully called out till they do command. There is nothing so invigorating, so inspiring, so regenerating. Everybody ought to obey. How delightful it is to obey some one who really knows what he is about, and can teach you—to learn, when one really feels that one is learning something. But let children speak and say how much they have learnt from their masters and their lessons.

Everybody ought, then, to command and to obey; and then we should hear no more of pride, and thinking much of oneself; for pride is the perversion of that desire of action which would then have found its proper exercise.

Great harm is done by striving after what is called "humility," by checking what is called "pride." It is a cry of nature to wish to be something—to do something. To check it is to check the appetite for activity which God has placed in our nature.

Humility is thinking meanly of ourselves, placing ourselves below others, and being willing that others should do so too.

Is not this rather absurdity and untruth? What I want is a true estimate of myself, not a false one. I want to see myself as God sees me. If a man with great physical strength were to say to one who has none, you are stronger than I, you can cut down that tree better than I: we should say "how wrong!" If Macaulay[11] were to persuade himself (for the sake of being humble) that he could not write history so well as any of the people at that moment walking down the Strand, would that be true or desirable? The maxim, let a man know what he can do, and do it, is not compatible with that of humility. Humility, if logically carried into our conduct, would lead to our giving up everything we do into the hands of those whom we are to strive to think can do it better than ourselves.

11. Thomas Babington Macaulay (1800–1859), English historian, essayist and statesman, and celebrated author of *The History of England* (5 vols., 1849–1861).

"Renouncing the world," would mean renouncing the great majority of mankind, of our fellow-men. Now mankind (or the world) is what we have to work upon. That we ought to seek the offices which we dislike most has no truth in it. Those who have an attraction, a fitness, (and these are many) for cooking and sweeping, ought to be sent to do it, not those who have a dislike to it. To "forget themselves and to despise the praises of men," the Catholics say. But the way to "forget yourself," (which is certainly of the first importance) is to be so much interested in some object out of yourself, that you can't remember yourself. If you are fully occupied, all your faculties in full and interesting exercise, you won't think about the praise of men.

Pride and conceit are not qualities either which will contribute to our oneness with God. But pride and conceit become impossible when we have a knowledge of the laws of God. If his laws have made me what I am, if without them I could not be what I am, and with them cannot be than what I am, how can I possibly be proud of what I am? They do away equally with pride and humiliation. The laws of God have brought me where I am. His laws will carry me through.

In "mortifying" ourselves to gain blessedness, in "humbling ourselves that we may be exalted," (though this is certainly founded on the words of Christ,) there is a good deal of the spirit of doing things for the sake of reward, and this, of course, is untrue and unhealthy.

There may be a pride even in humility, a self-seeking in suffering "abjection" (all pride is the effect of a narrowness of view), and therefore it is far safer not to be thinking about ourselves than to be seeking for "mortification."[12] Besides, it is ungrateful to God, when He is seeking to give you pleasure, always to take the worst—*not that some one else may have the best*, but only for the sake of mortifying your*self*, and especially, if you do this for the sake of having the best in another world.

To "renounce worldly enjoyment" implies a mistake. It should *be* our enjoyment to do the world's work.

It does not improve us to "hate" anything. One might easily excite oneself to hate all these luxuries. But it does us no good.

12. Nightingale elaborated on the idea of mortification in a letter (ca. 1853): "The mortification of the Sufi & the Fakir & the Derweesh was on a far more logical principle than the mortification of the R. Catholic or Puritan devotee—because they [Catholic and Puritan] were simply conjuring the anger of a passionate old Father—the Pantheistic Saint was not thinking of this, he was simply attaining the state of perfect happiness, which was to be, not given to him, but was itself indifference to the world, approach to or absorption in God by contemplation" (Claydon collection; *Calendar of Letters*, 3.C14,659).

The Catholics say that "through love of Christ's poverty the religious man should be glad when he has the poorest and worst things."

Surely it is a mistake to recommend poverty. Surely it is a higher pursuit to have property, in order that we may devote it to Him and do His work with it.

Christ was the most spiritual being who has ever lived. But surely he made mistakes. He is generally considered *either* as God or as an impostor. Now, much progress cannot be made unless we admit that he made mistakes, and we, Protestants, who profess to be the upholders of the Bible, do admit it practically, though we assert theoretically, that He was plenarily inspired, a man-God. What do boards of guardians make, for instance, of this his counsel of "poverty?" those who do not admit His wonderful spirituality cannot make much progress either. He was not a reasoner, certainly. For sometimes he speaks of leaving father and mother and lands as a sacrifice, and offers compensation elsewhere; and sometimes he tells us to hate them, and then it cannot be a sacrifice. He certainly was so indignant with the lukewarm spirit of the times, which was always making excuses, that he spoke in very strong words, "Let the dead bury their dead," "Hate your father and your mother," "Who is my mother and my brethren?"

The truth of the matter is probably that the attraction between husband and wife, and between all other friends should be this, that those two can do the work of God better together than apart, and then there would be no occasion to "leave them for His name's sake," but the contrary. When you have taken a wife, and undertaken the responsibility of children, *without* any such attraction, certainly there is no right in leaving them. With regard to leaving brothers and sisters, and father and mother, you have undertaken no charge with regard to them, and these should be left anyhow for God's work.

Men seem to think it will be pleasing to God that they should be ashamed of their human nature—they do not express sorrow that, endowed with a nature which has divine possibilities, they remain so poor: they prostrate themselves before the Source of all we are and all we might be, deploring their sinful nature—their impossibility to be or do anything that is right, except in as far as God works in and for them; and this is supposed to be humility pleasing to God. A just and true appreciation of what we are and what we may become, of how God will help us if we take the appointed means to receive His help, what He will do for us and what we are to do for ourselves, is the state which is true to our nature, true to God's nature. Pride is an aberration of mind, impossible except from misunderstanding of what we are, why we are, what we are to become. Self-satisfaction in humbling ourselves before God is misunderstanding as great in another direction. We can neither feel proud nor humble except from some misconception of God or of ourselves. If our state of mind is right, we shall press ever onward to be and to do in the infinite career before us. Such progress will be the want, the thirst of our nature—not undertaken to satisfy pride, not calling forth pride. To God we shall refer what we are, what we shall become, our means of becoming what it is fitting we should be. There will be no place in us where pride can enter. While the infinite is beyond, how can we feel proud of any step towards it?

V

A truly spiritual life, for Nightingale, is one in which all activities are organized so as to be in harmony with God's plan, that is, to facilitate the unfolding of the Divine within the human. Any type of work, even that which is considered menial, can thus serve a sacred purpose. She told Jowett in a letter that "it is a religious act to clean out a gutter and to prevent cholera, and that it is not a religious act to pray (in the sense of asking)."[13] She elaborated on this view in a private note entitled "Drains":

It is not the occupation but the spirit which makes the difference. The election of a bishop may be a most secular thing. The election of a representative may be a religious thing. It is not the preluding such an election with public prayer that would make it a religious act. It is religious so far as each man discharges his part as a duty and a solemn responsibility. The question is not whether a thing is done for the State or the Church, but whether it is done with God or without God.[14]

*   *   *

Will it be asked to what have we to trust to save human nature from falling into sin, if we give up the fear of God's anger if we sin? We have to trust to good feelings natural to man, which will *certainly* exist if we take the means to bring them into existence—means which would make it impossible to man to will wrong.

---

13. Letter dated 16 July 1862. Quoted in Quinn and Prest, *Dear Miss Nightingale*, p. 18.
14. Quoted in Cook, *Life of Florence Nightingale*, vol. 2, p. 240.

It may be said, "Look at this man and that. Are good feelings natural to them?—are they not lost, as far as we can see, to good feeling?"

If our physical nature is such that, fed and exercised in one way it would be strong, healthy, efficient to perform its functions; shall we, if it *is* fed in a different manner, say that man's frame is by nature weak and sickly?

We are often told that the heart of man is "desperately wicked, and deceitful above all things." Before accepting such doctrine, let us look to experience. Our feelings vary as they are exercised, as clearly, as certainly as the state of the physical nature varies with its food and exercise.

If the thoughts and feelings which befit a man are called forth, a human being will be *manly* in the true sense of the word. But many hearts are turned from their natural manliness, and will be so while man's life and circumstances do not afford to his nature its proper exercise.

But do we not see, it will be said, the truly great and good become greater and better in adverse circumstances?

It is most important, it is indeed essential, to discern what *are* adverse circumstances. In the first place, adverse to *what* do we mean? Those circumstances are really adverse to man, which impede in him the development and the exercise of the divine nature. It is said "such a man is in good circumstances," "is in easy circumstances." When we hear this, we know that it conventionally means, such a man has abundance of money. "He has ample means," signifies that he has an ample supply of money. But, whether the possession of money *is* equivalent to "good" or "easy" circumstances, or to "ample means" for attainment of the real object of life, opens up other questions, general and individual.

"It is easier for a camel to go through the eye of a needle than for a rich man to enter the kingdom of heaven" says the wisest and best of our instructors. Curious how many hear his words read as indisputable authority, yet habitually speak of riches as "easy circumstances." How little must we think of what we hear and accept as truth *or* of what we say!

But there are those who are rich *within*, whether, externally, they are rich or poor. Riches or poverty do not inevitably stand for favorable or unfavorable circumstances, as regards the development and exercise of the divine in man. What circumstances will develop it, what will strengthen it, what will afford it satisfaction,—this is the problem for the united efforts of man to solve, these are the circumstances for the united efforts of man to strive to effect. But no considerable portion of mankind have, as yet, had this problem distinctly before them, and there is little union in trying to discover it, or to realize it in life and work.

To get "money," or to use it as other people who have as much money usually do,—this occupies much of human life, employs much of human effort—some bestow their *surplus* of time and thought on divine objects and purposes. But there is not the *unity* which should make the *whole* of the object of the *whole* of mankind a search after the divine. This object would, no doubt, remain, in part, work for money. Money *may* facilitate the entrance into the "kingdom of heaven." Whether it will or not depends upon whether it becomes "ample means" to exercise a righteous nature.

It is so strange that life should be the only thing which we begin without having a type in our minds of what we mean it to be. We don't even build a house without seeing exactly before us that which we intend it should be when it is finished. We don't begin a drawing without knowing exactly what we mean to make of it; and *life*, which one would think the most important, is the only thing which people begin without any type or purpose at all before them.

It is God's purpose that man shall modify life and circumstances so that the outer world shall help the inner being to be one with God. Is man intent upon thus modifying circumstances? Till he is, trade may rise or fall, mines of gold lie hidden beneath the ground or millions lie scattered on its surface, there will be changes, without real progress, to mankind.

According to laws, not fathomed by us, nations will rise and fall. We shall vaguely ask the question, "Is England come to its culminating point?" as if there were a law that each nation was to rise and fall—not in accordance with any specific laws, but merely because the law was, rise and decline.

The religion of mankind is *without*, outside of them, making them discontented with themselves and their lives, whenever they think of it, but not helping them to improve their lives by themselves, themselves by their lives.

None of the great reformers have ever taken the way of life into account. Wesley—how much in earnest he was!—he preached and people were glad to hear. But did he say to the people, "Now while you are washing can you be in accordance with God?"

There must be washing, and ironing, and building, the earth must be cultivated; we must have food, and drink, and shelter. How can these occupations be organized so as to be in accordance with God's purpose instead of separating us from it?

Now we have not an idea of being in accordance with God's purpose. We put a great deal of food upon the table, but there is no thought of its being wholesome; there is no calculation of what will give us most strength and vigor to do God's work.

On the contrary, if we send for a physician we know that he will put us on a "regimen," and give us something quite different. The same as to dress; there is no thought of God's purpose. The same as to occupation.

Fashion directs us; *i.e.*, that which is conventional in our order.

Conventional life consists in this, in saying, "I am so sorry," "I hope you are coming," when we are not "sorry," and we do not "hope;" in *saying the proper thing without feeling it.* This is the first step in conventional life. The next step is when we actually do not know whether we feel it or not. And the last is when we have said what is "proper" till we do not know that we do not feel it—when we really think we feel a thing, because we have said it.

A true scheme for mankind would differ from all others in regard to this, that we should organize a *life* by which it would be possible to live in harmony with God's purpose. But now if we have been with Him in our "closet," we cease to be with Him as soon as we are at our work or with man, instead of being *more* with him when at our work, because it *His* work, and it is more in accordance with His purpose to work than to meditate. But there *is* now no purpose of this kind, and there never has been any purpose of this kind in any of the organizations or religions of nations. We have it set down in our minds that nations are to rise and fall; we make a little vague talk about "civilization" and "luxury;" but it is not set down in our minds that a nation living in disregard of God's purpose, when it comes to civilization and the enjoyments of civilization, must fall into selfish indulgence, thence into luxury, thence into decline and ruin.

"Whether ye eat or drink," says St. Paul, "do all to the glory of God." Does "good society" in England eat and drink "to the glory of God?" "Good society" in England acknowledges the Bible as inspired; a man is impeded in "society" if he is known to think otherwise. Yet, if one were to go to the highways of society, on its way to unwholesome and extravagant dinners, and speak forth these words, *that* one would be called a fanatic, and by the very men who would most strenuously oppose the admission into high offices of any one who said that the Bible was *not* peculiarly inspired, and that we are *not* bound to fashion our belief by it.

Such is our belief in this Book which we profess to believe. This is the most singular of all such states of mind, when people abandon that which they do care for, for that which they do not care for. Few care for the Church of England; yet men are sometimes seen giving up a friend whom they like because he does not belong to a Church to which they are indifferent.

Opinions on religion do not *now* model life. The habits of life are stamped in strong and durable fashion. That certain individuals, here and there, differ from orthodox views makes little impression on modes of life. Except in religious orders, the Roman Catholic, the Puseyite, the Evangelical, the Jew, in the higher and middle ranks of life, live much after the same fashion, though in different *coteries*, and refraining more or less from each other's society; but their habits do not differ materially or generally according to their religious views. If we study the varying manners of society (in our own country at least), we find them little influenced by religion. That which is called civilization in manners and habits, has it sprung from religion? Convenience and luxury advance from year to year; but does religion prompt them? The manners of the time of Sir Charles Grandison are very different from the manners of to-day. It would be amusing and interesting to spend a day among our ancestors of that date; but has religion influenced those changes? The Quakers speak and dress in certain formalisms, according to the directions of their religious ancestors. The Roman Catholics fast and attend to certain observances. But, generally speaking, is the way in which mankind employ themselves influenced by religion? Is their food, their dress, their conversation influenced by religion? Daily or weekly, on bended knees, at certain prescribed hours, to confess sins, little really felt or thought of—daily or weekly to offer praises and thanks to a Being little understood and little thought of—is not this the chief sign that religion exists at all in English society? In the time of Cromwell and among his followers, could we go back to spend a day with *them*, we should perhaps find a life really influenced by their views of religion; but where could we now track religion in life, *generally* speaking? Individuals will probably present themselves in each generation whose lives have sprung out of their religion; but not generations.

VI

Although Nightingale was critical of the narrow-mindedness found in many religious orders, she emphasized the importance of associations for the discovery of the true nature of religion and how it should be manifested in life. In her view, the discovery of truth is the result of the Divine Spirit acting within humanity. Truth is not miraculously given or revealed to one individual, independent of the whole, but is an evolutionary process requiring the united efforts of all mankind.

*   *   *

When we talk of the great realities of the universe, high wishes rise within us, we would strive to make our life divine. But, when we enter the petty details and purposes of our life, that divine spirit is aggrieved and sinks within us. To begin with, some few must unite in endeavouring to make life and work *one with* the divine thought and purpose, and, by degrees, humanity may become the working out of God's thought, which is its destination. At present it is indeed difficult to carry a true spirit into the details of life, such as life is. But we must strive to modify our life, as best we may, so as to keep alive the spirit of God within us.

Religious *life* and work require the healthy state and devotion of the spiritual, the affectional, the intellectual, and the physical nature. Each community of men should modify itself, and choose its chief leader and all subordinate leaders with a view to rendering its life and its work in accordance with the Spirit whence springs life.

We should aim at implicit obedience to leadership, together with scope for individual exercise of idiosyncracy—this is a difficult problem. The Perfect Spirit alone accomplishes it perfectly. His one Law of Truth and Right effects from every living being a perfect obedience. Yet each shall attain through it to the free exercise of his idiosyncracy. To fill up the practical detail of *how* such implicit obedience to government and such free exercise of idiosyncracy are to be attained in human government is a problem which ages must gradually solve. Certain it is that it must be the object of the human as well as the divine Governor in attaining implicit obedience to attain freedom for individual idiosyncracy. Hitherto, generally speaking, individual obedience checks freedom of idiosyncracy. But this is a remediable defect in the Governor and the governed, not one existing in the constitution of human nature.

In practice, all religious orders, both Protestant and Roman Catholic, fail in this. Each generally consists of one powerful mind at the head, and a great many childish minds under him (or her). If by chance another powerful mind creeps in among the subordinates, it throws all into confusion, it is called and *is* troublesome, and it ends by being expelled, expelling, or becoming stupefied.

In practice, religious orders never make progress. Great minds found them; little minds spring out of them. There is scarcely a historical instance of a discoverer, an inventor, a genius, or a benefactor of mankind being produced by a religious order *after* it is once compact and established. This is easily accounted for. There exists a certain personality, a want of interest in mankind *in general*, in the efforts of others,—a narrowness which leads the superior, who is (in theory and in reality) the moving spring, to think that his (still more her) own way is the only one for the world's salvation; that whatever does not spring from the same centre of thought is ruinous, and therefore to be discouraged; that the world, in fact, consists of himself (or herself), his (or her) community, and the poor immediately under their charge. There exists an impatience of interference (*all* other work being called by them "interference" with their own). This makes the usefulness of "orders" *per se* so narrow as to be nearly nugatory. I speak from experience. But the remark applies solely to those "orders" and "societies" which are not in constant official and essential contact with secular institutions. I speak quite as much of Protestant as of Roman Catholic "societies." The travelling "Sisters of Charity"[15] are perhaps the least stereotyped, the most exempt from this *exclusiveness,* which, where it exists, destroys all progress. The true "papacy," the real doctrine of "infallibility," exists in its complete-ness only in the *self*-constituted unchecked head of an "order," "society," parish, congregation, or doctrine.

Yet, while anxious to avoid the evils which experience has shown to arise in religious orders, we yet believe that *associations* with the object of discovering truth concerning the nature and will of God, the duty and nature of man—how to regulate life in accordance with such truth—are the probable, the natural means for causing mankind to advance in true belief, in true life. If two or three, or if one only, finds contradictions to the truth within him in the taught beliefs and in the ordinary lives of mankind, we would say to the few or the one, "Try to gain some few who would fervently wish to live as *one with God.*" But, if this is to be our endeavor, we must strive to know, and to declare to those few, the Being with whom we seek to be one. And here we may well imitate the best of the Roman Catholic orders, while on our guard against the evil incident to them. As with them, a fervently felt religion must be our bond. And, like the Roman Catholic orders, those who unite to seek a life springing from religion must unite in the reception of the same truth. We seek not to burn those who praise and worship, in God, what they would despise in man. We sympath-ize with parts of most religions. But if we unite together with a few to strive to live a life dictated by the Spirit of God, we must agree as to what that Spirit *is.* If *one* thinks it right to pray continually for forgiveness of sins, while another feels those sins to have been the cross which man bears for

15. More properly, the Daughters of Charity of Saint Vincent de Paul. The order was founded in France in 1633 by St. Vincent de Paul and St. Louise de Marillac, and was devoted to caring for the sick and the poor.

mankind, and that it is truth magnanimously to bear the cross of our past sins, while striving by God's means to emancipate ourselves and others from the burden of that cross—can these two be harmoniously, in life and feeling, one with God?

VII

What can we know of the Being we call God, but from the manifestation of His nature—His attributes? Look for His thought, His feeling, His purpose; in a word, His spirit within you, without you, behind you, before you. It is indeed omnipresent. Work your true work, and you will find His presence in your self—*i.e.*, the presence of those attributes, those qualities, that spirit, which is all we know of God. If we recognise this spirit without us in the rule of the universe—if we recognise this spirit within us, whenever man is well at work, may we not say "He is in us, and we in Him?"

We shall find this no vain or fanciful theory. If we seek Him by true work, true life, we shall find Him (*i.e.*, His attributes which are all we know of Him) within us; limited indeed, as is right, till our life and work shall attain for us higher regions of being—*i.e.*, greater love, greater wisdom, greater power.

Well it is that power is so limited, while love and wisdom are so feeble. Blessed are the limits of humanity, till it has advanced to greater purity and truth! Peculiar power, whether arising from nature or from circumstances, is seldom now a good for the individual or for mankind.

And let all this be tested by the realities of life, striving to look at these comprehensively, in relation to all being and all successions of being. Thus only can we, in any degree, see as God sees, which is "truth."

*   *   *

In her classic work on mysticism, Evelyn Underhill wrote that "true mysticism is active and practical, not passive and theoretical."[16] This characteristic aptly describes Nightingale's approach to the spiritual life, which emphasizes a unity with God achieved through "deeds, not creeds." This active element might have been an Unitarian influence,

16. Evelyn Underhill, *Mysticism: A Study in the Nature and Development of Man's Spiritual Consciousness*, p. 81.

but should also be viewed as a logical extension of her idea that by working our "true work," we find the "heaven within." This concept is not unlike that of *dharma* in Hinduism and Buddhism; the latter in one sense denotes activities or duties specifically suited for individuals, by which one contributes to and participates in cosmic order, and is thus led into a state of spiritual bliss. In her copy of Sir Edwin Arnold's *Song Celestial* (translation of the Indian *Bhagavad-Gita*), Nightingale marked the following passage:

> Abstaining from attachment to the work,
> Abstaining from rewardment in the work,
> While yet, one doeth it faithfully,
> Saying, "Tis right to do!"—that is true act
> And abstinence! Who doeth duties so,
> Unvexed if his work fail, if it succeed
> Unflattered, in his own heart justified,
> Quit of debates and doubts, his is "true" act.[17] (XVIII, 9–10)

*   *   *

"Thy kingdom come." If we seek Christ's most abiding, his uppermost thought, it was this. And what did Christ understand by "Thy kingdom?" He explains in those memorable words, "the kingdom of God is within you." There are no more satisfactory words of His. How much is contained in them! Earth *may* be heaven. But man is of the earth now, and there are so many good and pleasant things now rife in life that man is particularly liable to forget how great he might be—to be satisfied with being an amused and amusing child. Let him arouse himself to a consciousness of the divine within him, as pleasant and cheerful days pass among those around him. It was to the poor the Gospel was preached. And, if another Christ came to draw fresh supplies from the well of truth which fails not, he would still speak to the poor. Truth is a *speculation* among the rich. Among the poor, there might be a few who would listen and care to find more truth in life than it now manifests. We must be patient, but never failing in fervour for God's work, ready to work and, which is much harder, ready to wait. Then may some seed be sown in this world, and we may be learning for other spheres, when we cannot learn for this.

17. Quoted in Cook, *Life of Florence Nightingale*, vol. 2, p. 242.

7. On Life After Death

There is nothing final in the universe of mind or of matter—all is tendency, growth.

I

Nightingale's philosophy revolved around a Spirit of Right, a Perfect Being possessing a wise and benevolent will. She was therefore compelled, like the great minds throughout the ages, to formulate an eschatology that did not contradict her concept of God. She never seems to have had a morbid attitude toward death, always regarding it as an integral part of the divine plan. As a young woman of twenty-six, she wrote:

I cannot pretend to speak of death as a misfortune . . . Death is the arch of triumph under which the soul passes to live again in a purer and freer atmosphere.[1]

During her travels through Egypt, she was confronted by an ancient culture that commemorated the dead with enduring monuments on an unparalleled scale. Her efforts to grasp a sense of of the ancients' attitudes toward death seemed to help in articulating her own beliefs:

I have often thought there was much more evidence for a future world than there is for this. For the existence of this [world], we can only draw evidence from our perception . . . for the existence of another, we can draw evidence from our reason, our feeling, our consciousness . . . But the Egyptians seem to have gone farther; they seem to have said, we will consider this life as interesting only in its connection with the whole of which it is a part. I have often thought how dull we were not to see that Christ's life *showed* us this more advanced stage of existence which we call heaven; how we have persisted in

1. *Calendar of Letters*, 2.A9,282.

calling him the "man of sorrows," instead of calling him the man who is already in a state of blessedness, the man who has progressed and succeeded.[2]

Despite her outlook, she never became cavalier about death and spent the rest of her life trying to improve public health and end suffering. After the Crimean War, she was haunted by the memories of the fallen soldiers whose deaths might have been prevented with adequate supplies and facilities.

For Nightingale the question of death was relatively simple: as each individual embodies unique qualities that cannot be duplicated, it would not be consistent with God's benevolent nature to obliterate that being. Because it is God's plan to raise mankind from imperfection to perfection, death must initiate a different mode of existence, one that allows for continued development.

*   *   *

Whence does the question arise, whether human consciousness will be continued after the existence of man, such as he is in this world? The plant withers and dies: we never think of asking whether there will be any continuation of its individuality; we are satisfied with observing that matter never ceases to exist, but only changes from one mode of existence to another. Of this the senses assure all who attend to the subject.

But very many are not satisfied to take it for granted that, when man dies, the change in his material form is the only result. The heart which has loved and sympathized, revered and admired, asks, "Is this dust all that remains from qualities of the same nature as those to be recognized in the Perfect?" The heart which has watched suffering asks, when in vain trying to relieve it, "Is there no relief but unconsciousness?" Still more, the heart which mourns over a vicious existence, conscious that, if this be all, for this man it would be better that he had never been born, since his existence is not worth having; yet, conscious also that he had no power to make it otherwise, asks whether there may not be future opportunity in which the experience of the past may lead to a better future? The capabilities of the nature of the plant are fulfilled; but man, to whose capabilities none can put a limit in themselves—man, full of high object, making discoveries, or

2. *Letters from Egypt,* p. 74.

otherwise exercising his faculties, so that his life is enriching mankind! Is he to share the fate of the plant?

But he bequeaths, it is said, the riches of his nature to posterity, when he himself becomes insensible dust.

Each individual is an idiosyncratic nature, different from every other that is, or has been or ever will be. It is impossible that he should communicate all that he is, all that he has to communicate, except through himself. Whatever the possibilities of his nature, it is by *exercise* only that he can realize or communicate them. To his power of attainment or of communication it does not seem that there is any necessary close before death. Many live to old age, in healthy possession of their faculties till death. That many do not, is owing to mistakes in the mode of life. The affection which any one feels for another, whose life he has shared, can never be repeated by any other. Fresh affections may arise between individuals of fresh generations. But can succession equal, in kind or degree, continuity? During the space of a brief human life, what is there not to do? There is to prepare the nature for such attachments, to find out, by the experience of actual life, the persons capable of being mutually inspired with them; there are the mistakes to be made; each other's characters to be felt after in the dark; and heart-aches from having misunderstood, or not adapted ourselves to the characters we are attached to.

But, granting that, each generation transmitting its experience, man will arrive at exemption from such mistakes; that, by dint of this experience transmitted by one generation to another, he will attain to a well-constituted nature, to good means of cultivating and exercising it, to a good organization of life, so that the most will be made of life, and thus that opportunity will not be lost by mistakes.

But then still more will it be felt that the ties of sympathy, of capability of communicating mutually, between any two, are different from what can be between any other two—that to put an end to such ties would be to destroy that which, by the laws of God, can never be again. Such destruction of that which is valuable—of that which can never be renewed, would not be consistent with the existence of an omnipresent spirit of love and wisdom.

It *has* been thought right, in some stages of society, to compel one man to sacrifice himself for others, but experience teaches us that, whether our object be selfish or benevolent, it is not, in the nature of things, to be gained by sacrificing one for another. It is impossible indeed to sacrifice one for another, if we would. That which is good for all is essentially good for each. That which is bad for one is bad for all. It would, therefore, be bad for all, a loss to all that any individual nature were put out of existence; for each individual nature has a capability of contributing to the whole, in a way that no other nature can.

To suppose that each individual does contribute his portion, and then retires from existence to make room for others, is inconsistent with the hypotheses of a spirit of love and wisdom, *i.e.*, such a Being would not bring into existence a capability which, from the nature of things, no other will have, and then destroy that capability. It is true that *something* is transmitted to another generation; but experience shows that no mode of existence is wasted or destroyed. It is all evolution, development, order, progress,—never destruction.

But to this it is answered that a human being does *not* cease to exist at death. It is change, not destruction, which takes place.

Do you mean the change from a human being to dust and gases? Think what a human being is, think of the divine nature existing in kind, only limited in degree, and say if you can think dust and gases the development, the evolution, to a human being in the thought of the omnipotent spirit of love and goodness?

Is it not obvious, too, that the physical being exists, as the means or mode for the existence of the divine attributes, for the attainment of them by exercise, for their exercise when attained?

The physical being is the *means*,—the divine nature, or the attainment and exercise of the divine nature, the *end*.

By observation and experience we trace that God makes the right exercise of the collective nature of mankind, the means and measure of the well-being of the individual and the race. And we find, by experience and observation, that this must be the means and measure of man's benefit to man—that one man *can* only help another by helping him to some right exercise of his own nature. Having discovered this, we may infer that God will not destroy, when attained by exercise, that which can only, agreeably to His purpose, be thus attained.

Granted that every material argument is against a future existence, that it is impossible to believe memory continued where the system of physical relations is changed—then we depend simply and solely upon moral evidence, upon the moral character of God, for our belief in a future state.

And this is thought a very poor dependence. Certainly, we have no other. But *whatever* co-existences or successions are observable, the only fundamental source of all or any of them is the will of the spirit of right. We ask, "Is *this* possible? is *that* possible?" The fundamental question is, "Is *this* or *that* consistent with God, the spirit of right?" We are apt to think that those co-existences, which we believe to be invariable, arise from some connexion in their *own* nature, but their nature springs from the will of the ruling spirit of right, from no other source.

With regard to a continuation of this existence, it is not, as respects ourselves or our friends, any eagerness for the enjoyment of life, any repugnance to the idea as respects ourselves or them, of ceasing to exist; but a desire to be convinced that there is a continued existence for each identity, *because* such a conviction alone accords with our idea of what is right in the supreme will.

It is true, however, that we have no real "foundation" but "faith" for believing in a future life.

We are told that faith will remove mountains. It has been supposed that the more contrary to the usual course of things, the greater the miracle, the greater the power manifested by God, the greater is our merit in believing in His power. But, if the mountain is stable through God's law, shall we conceive Him to exercise His power in violating that law? Christ seemed to conceive that a man would be empowered to do whatever he believed that he could do,—but would there be any right in such a principle as this?

Yet faith will remove all the difficulties which, we acknowledge, lie in the way of believing in a future state. What is faith?* Is it belief that God will break his own laws, that he will vary from the nature whence they spring? No, it is belief that his nature, and consequently his laws, are invariable. He has given us the means to recognize what goodness and benevolence, and righteousness, and wisdom are. Men have varied, indeed,

---

*The following passages are from Mackay's "Progress of the Intellect:"

"In its advanced stages, faith is a legitimate result of the calculation of probabilities; it may transcend experience, but can never absolutely contradict it. Faith and knowledge tend mutually to the confirmation and enlargement of one another; faith by verification being often transformed into knowledge, and every increase of knowledge supplying a wider and firmer basis of belief. Faith, as an inference from kowledge, should be consistently inferred from the whole of knowledge."

"The same experience which is the source of knowledge being therefore the only legitimate foundation of faith, a sound faith cannot be derived from the anomalous and exceptional. It is the avidity for the marvellous, and the morbid eagerness for a cheap and easy solution of the mysteries of existence, a solution supposed to be implied in the conception of an arbitrary and unintelligible rule, which has ever retarded philosophy and stultified religion. Faith naturally arises out of the regular and undeviating. The same unerring uniformity which alone makes experience possible, was also the first teacher of the invisible things of God."

and do vary, as to their conceptions of what these are. So they have done, and do, concerning other truths, which are yet within human ken. But on every subject there is a truth; and unity of opinion will come just in proportion as mankind gain knowledge of truth and improvement of being.

II

Although she is unclear about the nature of life after death, Nightingale implies that the developmental process is cyclical in nature: the individual merges with the Divine, but "then again sets forth to work and live, and manifest, and realize fresh phases of being." This concept of cyclic manifestation is suggestive of reincarnation, a belief with which Nightingale was acquainted through her studies of Plato, particularly the *Phaedo* and the *Republic*, Book X. In her letters from Egypt, she discussed the belief in reincarnation among the ancient pharaohs, quoting Plato as her source:

If they are but ordinary beings, I believe Plato thinks that 10,000 years will be the time before they come again. But at the end of every 1000 years, they will be able to choose what life they will have next; and upon this choice depends much of what they would become . . . And if I were a Pharaoh now, I would choose the Arab form, and come back to help these poor people; and I am going tomorrow to a tomb of a Rameses, 1150 B.C. to meet him and tell him so.[3]

She also spoke of reincarnation in an essay appended to her letters from Egypt, entitled "Vision of Temples."[4] In this fictional tale inspired by her visits to the ancient temples, she described how after "centuries of purification" the spirits of Egyptian kings returned to look upon their monuments. Lacking a true understanding of the nature of God, the kings are reincarnated to increase their wisdom and insight.

Ideas consistent with a belief in reincarnation were shared by many of Nightingale's contemporaries, including William Wordsworth, Samuel Coleridge, Robert Browning, Alfred Tennyson, and Matthew Arnold, as well as her one-time suitor Richard Monckton Milnes and her good

3. *Letters from Egypt*, pp. 133–134.
4. "Vision of Temples" did not appear in Anthony Sattin's edition of *Letters from Egypt*.

friend and secretary A. H. Clough.[5] Max Müller was particularly instrumental in introducing such concepts to the west by means of his translations of Indian scriptures. He himself embraced the idea of reincarnation, and wrote:

I cannot help thinking that the souls towards whom we feel drawn in this life are the very souls whom we knew and loved in the former life, and the souls who repel us here we do not know why, are the souls that earned our disapproval, the souls from whom we kept aloof in a former life.[6]

*   *   *

Perhaps increased knowledge of the nature of God may reveal to us that each present mode of being is part of a development from a past without beginning, towards a future without end; all *except* the one eternal Spirit, whose thought, whose feeling, whose purpose, whose will, comprehends every other mode of being.

The subject of *Individualism*, if better understood, would throw great light upon this. Does that which is individual in thought and feeling always remain individual? or does it remain individual till, through progress attained, it merges in the one all-comprehensive nature, carrying to it its phase of thought and feeling, made concrete in life, manifested in activity, in work? Was there never a time when the spirit of love, of wisdom, of truth, of righteousness, did not exist? What is time? All that we know of it is succession of events. And is there any reason within or without us for supposing that this spirit in any succession of events did not exist? in any succession of events will not exist? And if the thought, the sentiment of right, and love, and wisdom is eternal, will not its manifestation in life, in activity, be eternal?

And will this manifestation be an eternal development or an eternal succession? Development carries the past into the future; succession begins where the past has left off. The smallest seed which develops into a plant, carries on into that plant the nature of every seed which preceded it. The elective king or ruler takes up circumstances where his predecessor laid them down. In him is not development. The thought, the feeling, the character of man, is by far the most interesting mode of existence of which

5. See Joseph Head and S. L. Cranston, comps., *Reincarnation: An East-West Anthology.*
6. *Reincarnation*, p. 160.

we have any knowledge or conception, except the thought, the feeling, the character of God.

Development from one individual thought, feeling, character to another, cannot take place by succession, by one character taking up circumstances where another left them.

Hence, perceiving development to be God's mode of proceeding, we are led to expect development from one state of character into another.

Dr. Priestley[7] came to the conclusion that the laws of material existence would prove that man ceases to exist at death but for revelation, in which he was so firm a believer, that his confidence in a future life appears to have been as strong as his consciousness of a present one.

We believe with him that the laws of physical existence all teach that death is the end of human existence; but the revelation which proves the contrary is not made by God through miraculously inspired teachers; it is a revelation made by the various capabilities of observing and reflecting, of thinking and feeling, which God has given to mankind.

Is it asked, what beings will live after this life ceases? Every mode of being which admits of thought and feeling; for such modes of being require eternity for their development. No thought, no feeling, can have attained perfection, can have acted and lived perfection, in any limited period. Each individual thinking, feeling being, by the law of the Perfect, works upward, directly or indirectly,—attains to the perfect thought and feeling which comprehends all, which feels and wills all truth,—and then again sets forth to work and live, and manifest, and realize fresh phases of being, guided by the law of the all-comprehensive spirit.

Now every present influences the character as an individuality. May we believe that each character is, and will remain, an individuality through eternity? Or must we suppose that the individuality goes on till, by progress, worked out by exercise, all knowledge is attained—till God's thought, which is the revelation of knowledge present, past, and future, is attained—and then His being is shared, His purpose is shared, viz., that of turning a fresh phase of purpose into life, exercise, work? But, then, will this bring to an end individual affections? Not necessarily; for the Perfect thus contains in His nature all the individual affections which ever were, matured by life and work, in one. And this one, in again individualizing, according to the laws of righteousness and benevolence, contains in its nature those same individuals which may again meet as individuals, again merge into perfec-

7. Joseph Priestley (see Introduction, p. xxi).

tion—perfection of thought and feeling, now and for ever, but such thought and feeling ever anew worked out in successive phases of life.

This is not pantheism, which asserts that man will be merged in God and lose his individuality.

"The spirit returns to God who gave it" *is* pantheism. And this cannot be true in the sense that it ceases to have a separate existence. Why, in that case, its trials? Can we suppose that God sent forth a being to suffer and struggle, merely in order that it should be re-absorbed into God's existence. Most lame and impotent conclusion. Why send it forth? To what end its suffering?

Individuality appears to be sacred in the thought of God. Indeed, if we suppose man to be a modification of the attributes of God limited by the laws of physical nature, it seems natural to expect that individuality will be preserved in every instance till perfection is attained.

It is obvious that the tendency of the right exercise of man's capabilities is towards perfection. In whatever direction he *wisely* exercises his faculties he improves, and in no direction has come into view the point at which improvement must stop, except indeed improvement in physical power. A man may improve in physical strength up to a certain point, but he cannot even keep up permanently to that point, much less go beyond it. But it would seem that experience already gives prospect of endless improvement in various intellectual and moral directions, *infinite* prospect of removing ignorance and inability.

Let it be remembered that happiness will be best promoted, not by exercise of skill and ability in a certain direction, irrelative to one general object to which all exercise of human nature should tend, viz., order, progress, living for others in accordance with the thought of righteousness, goodness, wisdom—happiness will be best promoted by each exercising himself according to his own individual nature so as to contribute to the purpose common to all.

Both the highest and the lowest human natures, then, lead to the same conclusion, viz., a future state of infinite progress for each and for all. The higher natures, in proportion as they are high, teach that the spirit of perfect, omnipotent love and wisdom will never destroy that which is of highest value, which by the laws of the Perfect can never be replaced. The lower natures, in proportion as they are low, teach that there is a future through which that existence which is not now a boon will become so, otherwise such existence would not be consistent with the will from which it springs.

Our real, practical reason for believing in a future life is the same that men believe upon and act upon throughout their practical life, viz.:—that *will* will correspond with the nature of the character whence it springs, and that that nature exists in accordance with some law or principle. Why do I depend on finding my meal prepared this morning? on meeting my friend at noon? on finding the committee collected which I expect this afternoon? Is it not all dependence upon will, upon the nature whence will springs? I find it to be essential to will to pursue its greatest satisfaction, or, in other words, I find that, essentially, it does not *dis*-satisfy itself. I can give no mathematical proof that, at nine o'clock, I shall find breakfast on the table,—at three I shall find collected a committee for a particular purpose. But I no more doubt it than I doubt the existence of the pen and ink which I see before me.

Once assured that there exists a *will*, whence spring the successive phenomena or modes of existence in the universe; once convinced that the nature of that will is the same benevolence and wisdom of which I am conscious in human nature,—and I depend on a continuation of existence. Because the Omnipotent willing otherwise would contradict the benevolence and wisdom which His universe reveals.

If you will strive to observe, study and comprehensively interpret the universe in its eternal purport, you will discern more and more one will, one nature, upon which you may depend. You could not bring yourself to conceive that your friends in this house would leave you this morning without your daily meal. Stretch your thought to the revelations of the universe, and still less will you feel it a possibility that God will quench the spirit than that man will starve the body.

The more, in ages to come, mankind shall become convinced, by the evil actually remedied by man, of human possibility to remedy all evil—of human possibility to progress in righteousness and knowledge by progress actually made—the more the experience how each existing character can help the human family as no other can—the stronger will become the conviction that each individuality is intended to help God's family in the universe after, as well as during, his present phase of being. Hence, without increased means of conceiving the mode of existence after death, human belief in it may be strengthened.

The ceaseless change which goes on through all existence except One, whose will directs it, is all development—all the fulfilling of purpose. Time, in one sense, is as nothing to the eternal One. He will realize the full, the perfect development which is His thought, though it require ages beyond the grasp of our minds to conceive.

Appendix 1. Guide to the Text

This edition of *Suggestions for Thought* represents a major reorganization of the original material. The following table indicates the locations in the original three volumes for most of the passages we have chosen.

Chapter 1, "On the Concept of God"

section I:	vol. 1: pp. 6–7, 42–43, 180
	vol. 2: pp. 5, 38, 111–113, 192–195
section II:	vol. 2: pp. 306–312
section III:	vol. 1: pp. 3–5, 13–16, 219
	vol. 2: pp. 139–140
section IV:	vol. 1: pp. 25, 49–52, 198–199
	vol. 2: pp. 82–84, 94, 102, 181–183
	vol. 3: p. 68
section V:	vol. 1: pp. 50, 301–303
	vol. 2: pp. 40–41, 97, 293–300

Chapter 2, "On Universal Law"

section I:	vol. 1: pp. 43–45,
section II:	vol. 1: pp. 26–27, 137, 144–146, 184–185, 229–230
	vol. 3: pp. 6–7
section III:	vol. 2: pp. 16–17, 48–51
section IV:	vol. 2: pp. 98–101, 113–118, 145–146, 304, 310–311
	vol. 3: pp. 46–47
section V:	vol. 1: pp. 39–41
	vol. 2: pp. 86–88, 161–163
	vol. 3: pp. 62–63

Chapter 3, "On God's Law and Human Will"

section I:	vol. 1: p. 71
section II:	vol. 1: pp. 247–248, 261–262, 267–271
	vol. 2: pp. 201–203
	vol. 3: pp. 55, 75
section III:	vol. 1: pp. 72–73, 75–76, 136–138, 141–142
	vol. 3: p. 54
section IV:	vol. 1: pp. 142–144, 150–151, 204
	vol. 3: pp. 49–50, 52–53
section V:	vol. 1: pp. 147–149, 151, 155–156

Chapter 4, "On Sin and Evil"

section I: vol. 1: pp. 12–13, 67, 69–70
section II: vol. 1: pp. 78–88, 94–96
section III: vol. 1: pp. 232–233
                    vol. 2: pp. 6–8
                    vol. 3: pp. 71–72, 78
section IV: vol. 2: pp. 208–211
section V: vol. 2: pp. 349–351
                    vol. 3: pp. 68–71

Chapter 5: "On Family Life"

section I: vol. 2: pp. 386–387, 394 ("Cassandra")
section II: vol. 2: pp. 197–200, 276–277, 389 ("Cassandra")
section III: vol. 2: pp. 219–224
section IV: vol. 2: pp. 64–70, 380 ("Cassandra")
section V: vol. 2: pp. 404, 408–410 ("Cassandra")

Chapter 6, "On the Spiritual Life"

section I: vol. 1: pp. 65–66, 101–102, 159–162
                    vol. 2: pp. 108, 346
section II: vol. 1: pp. 56–58, 60–61
section III: vol. 1: pp. 163–164
                    vol. 2: pp. 19–22, 24, 26, 28–35, 45–46, 164–166, 316–317, 322
section IV: vol. 2: pp. 23, 46–47, 128, 153–154
                    vol. 3: pp. 82–83
section V: vol. 2: pp. 54–55, 108–110
                    vol. 3: p. 66, 79–81
section VI: vol. 2: pp. 328–330, 350
section VII: vol. 2: pp. 85, 315–316

Chapter 7, "On Life After Death"

section I: vol. 1: pp. 106–110, 112–113, 115–117
section II: vol. 1: pp. 82, 121–124
                    vol. 3: pp. 111–112, 115, 120

Appendix 2. Chronology

As noted in the Introduction, the next few pages provide a chronological reference for the text. Significant events in Nightingale's life appear on the right, contemporary events on the left.

CONTEMPORARY EVENTS

1825–26   J. H. Newman's *Miracles of Scripture*.

1827   E. B. Pusey's *An Historical Enquiry into the Probable Causes of the Rationalist Character Lately Predominant in the Theology of Germany*.

1828   The Test and Corporation Acts are repealed, thereby allowing dissenters to hold public office.

1829   The Catholic Emancipation Act is passed, thereby allowing Catholics to hold public office.

1833   The Oxford Movement begins.
Institution of Deaconesses founded at Kaiserswerth.

1834   Connop Thirlwall is dismissed from Cambridge for advocating the admission of dissenters to the university.

1835   David Friedrich Strauss's *Das Leben Jesu*.

1836   James Martineau's *The Rationale of Religious Enquiry*.

1837   Queen Victoria begins her reign.

1838   F. D. Maurice's *The Kingdom of Christ*.
University of London opens to all men "without distinction."

1841   J. H. Newman's *Tract XC*.
Christian von Bunsen appointed Prussian envoy to England.
Joint Anglo-Prussian bishopric established in Jerusalem.
Quetelet organizes the Commission Central de Statistique in Belgium.

1842   J. S. Mill's *A System of Logic*.
J. H. Newman's *Miracles of Early Ecclesiastical History*.

1845   J. H. Newman converts to Roman Catholicism.
Anglican Sisters of the Holy Cross founded.

1846   F. Max Müller arrives in England.
Strauss's *Das Leben Jesu* translated by George Eliot.

1847   The "Gorham Case" begins.

1848   Cholera epidemic (1848–49).
Lydia Priscilla Sellon establishes the Sisterhood of Mercy.

1849   Max Müller's translation of the *Rigveda* is published.
J. A. Froude's *Nemesis of Faith*.

NIGHTINGALE'S LIFE AND WORK

1820   Born in Florence, Italy.

1837   Experiences her first "call" from God. Nightingale family embarks on European tour (1837–39), during which Florence meets Mary Clarke and Julius Mohl.

1842   Meets Christian von Bunsen.

1846   Receives the Yearbook of the Institution of Deaconesses from Bunsen.

1847–48   Travels to Italy where she meets Sidney Herbert, Henry Manning, and Mary Stanley. Goes on retreat at the convent Trinità dei Monte.

1849–50   Travels to Egypt, where God "speaks" to her, and to Greece. Visits Kaiserswerth before returning home.

1850   Privy Council rules in favor of Gorham.
        Henry Manning converts to Roman Catholicism.

1851   Religious census taken.

1853   F. D. Maurice is forced to resign from King's College after the publication
        of his *Theological Essays*.
        Cholera epidemic (1853–54).
        International Statistical Congress founded.
        Comte's *Cours de philosophie positive* translated by Harriet Martineau.

1854   Crimean War begins.
        Bunsen resigns his diplomatic post and returns to Germany.
        Baden Powell's *The Order of Nature*.
        Dissenters admitted to Oxford.

1855   Benjamin Jowett's *Epistles of St. Paul*. Vice-chancellor of Oxford asks him to
        resubscribe to the Thirty-Nine Articles.

1856   Treaty of Paris ends the Crimean War.
        Rowland Williams's *Christianity and Hinduism*.
        Dissenters admitted to Cambridge.

1858   Jews admitted to Parliament.
        "Great Stink" in London caused by sewage in Thames.

1859   Darwin's *The Origin of Species*.
        John Stuart Mill's *On Liberty*.

1860   The Broad Church's *Essays and Reviews*.
        Baron von Bunsen dies in Germany.

1861   Sidney Herbert, A. H. Clough, and Prince Albert die.

1862   H. B. Wilson and R. Williams tried for heresy and acquitted.

1863   Bishop J. W. Colenso (South Africa) deposed for pointing out biblical
        inconsistencies in his *Pentateuch Criticially Examined*.
        B. Jowett charged with heresy but acquitted.

1851   Spends 3 months at Kaiserswerth while her mother attends Parthenope at Carlsbad.
Begins *Suggestions for Thought* (?)

1852   Considers converting to Roman Catholicism.
Writes *Cassandra* and prepares proof for *Suggestions for Thought*.

1853   Attempts on several occasions to spend time at the hospital of the Sisters of Charity in Paris.
Appointed superintendent of the Institution for the Care of Sick Gentlewomen in Distressed Circumstances.

1854–56   Serves as Superintendent of Nurses in the British army hospitals in the Crimea.

1857   Royal Commission on the Health of the Army is established under her influence.

1858   *Notes on Matters Affecting the Health, Efficiency and Hospital Administration of the British Army.*
Arthur H. Clough becomes Nightingale's secretary.

1859   *Notes on Hospitals.* Royal Commission on the Health of the British Army in India is established.

1860   *Notes on Nursing.*
Suggestions for Thought is privately printed. Friendship with Benjamin Jowett ensues.
The Nightingale Training School for Nurses is established.

1861   King's College Training Scool for Midwives is established.
Asked by the American Secretary of War for assistance in organizing army hospitals for casualities of the Civil War.

1863   Publishes article on the Contagious Diseases Act.
Observations on the evidence contained in the stational returns for the Royal Commission on the Sanitary State of the Army in India.
How People May live and Not Die in India.

1864   Contagious Diseases Act passed.
       Newman's *Apologia Pro Vita Sua.*

1865   J. B. Mozley's *Eight Lectures on Miracles.*

1866   Last major cholera epidemic.
       J. S. Mill presents women's suffrage petition to Parliament.

1869   J. S. Mill's *The Subjection of Women.*
       Vatican Council I (1869–70).

1871   Universities' Test Act passed, thereby eliminating religious tests as a re-
       quirement to matriculation and graduation.

1873   Jowett's *The School and Children's Bible.*

1874   London Medical College for Women established.

1876   Julius von Mohl dies.

1878   Degrees at University of London opened to women.
       Women admitted to lectures at Oxford.

1882   British occupy Cairo to quell revolt.

1883   Mary Clarke Mohl dies.

1886   Contagious Diseases Act is repealed.

1887   Celebration of Queen Victoria's Golden Jubilee.

1893   B. Jowett dies.

1897   Celebration of Victoria's Diamond Jubilee.

1901   Death of Queen Victoria.

1864   *Suggestions in regard to Sanitary Works required for the Improvement of Indian Stations.*

1865   *Suggestions on a system of nursing for hospitals in India.*

1867   Organizes Sanitary Commission of India Office.
       Suggestions on the subject of providing training, and organizing nurses for the sick poor in workhouse infirmaries.

1868   *Method of improving the nursing service of hospitals.*

1870   Serves as advisor to French and Prussian army medical service during Franco-Prussian War.
       Supervises activities of the National Society for Aid to the Sick and Wounded.

1871   *Introductory notes on lying-in institutions.*

1872   Assists Jowett with translations of Plato.
       Selects stories for Children's Bible.

1873   Writes two articles on theological subjects for *Fraser's Magazine*.
       Begins work on *Notes From Devotional Authors of the Middle Ages*.

1874   W. E. Nightingale dies.

1880   Fanny Nightingale dies.

1882   Organizes team of nurses to serve during Egyptian campaign: "It is the Crimea over again."

1887   Notes her "Jubilee" year: fifty years since God first called her to His service.

1890   Parthenope dies.

1894   Sir Harry Verney, Parthenope's husband, dies.

1907   Receives the Order of Merit from King Edward VII.

1910   Dies at age 90.

Bibliography

Works by and about Florence Nightingale

Allen, Donald R. "Florence Nightingale: Toward a Psychohistorical Interpretation." *Journal of Interdisciplinary History* 6, 1 (Summer 1975): 23–45.

Bishop, William John and Sue Goldie, comps. *A Bio-Bibliography of Florence Nightingale*. London: Dawsons of Pall Mall, 1962.

Boyd, Nancy. *Three Victorian Women Who Changed Their World: Josephine Butler, Octavia Hill, Florence Nightingale*. New York: Oxford University Press, 1982.

Brook, Marion J. "Some Thoughts and Reflections on the Life of Florence Nightingale from a Twentieth Century Perspective." In Bullough et al., eds., *Florence Nightingale and Her Era: A Collection of New Scholarship*, pp. 23–29.

Bullough, Vern, Bonnie Bullough, and Marietta P. Stanton, eds. *Florence Nightingale and Her Era: A Collection of New Scholarship*. New York: Garland, 1990.

Calabria, Michael D. "Spiritual Insights of Florence Nightingale." *The Quest* 3, 2 (Summer 1990): 66–74.

Cohen, I. Bernard. "Florence Nightingale." *Scientific American* 250, 3 (March 1984): 128–37.

Cook, Sir Edward Tyas. *The Life of Florence Nightingale*. 2 vols. New York: Macmillan, 1913. Reprint 1942.

"Florence Nightingale as a Leader in the Religious and Civic Thought of Her Time." *Hospitals* 10 (July 1936): 78–84.

Goldie, Sue. *A Calendar of the Letters of Florence Nightingale*. Oxford: Oxford Microform Publications, 1983.

Huxley, Elspeth. *Florence Nightingale*. New York: G. P. Putnam's Sons, 1975.

Keele, Mary, ed. *Florence Nightingale in Rome: Letters Written by Florence Nightingale in Rome in the Winter of 1847–1848*. Memoirs of the American Philosophical Society 143. Philadelphia: American Philosophical Society, 1981.

Mantripp, J. C. "Florence Nightingale and Religion." *London Quarterly Review* 157 (July 1932): 318–25.

Nightingale, Florence. *Cassandra: An Essay*. Edited by Myra Staik with an epilogue by Cyntha McDonald. Old Westbury, NY: Feminist Press, 1979.

———. *Cassandra and Other Selections from Suggestions from Thought*. Edited by Mary Poovey. NYU Press Women's Classics. New York: New York University Press, 1992.

———. *Letters from Egypt*. London: A & G.A. Spottiswoode, 1854.

———. *Letters from Egypt: A Journey on the Nile, 1849–1850.* Selected and with an introduction by Anthony Sattin. New York: Weidenfeld and Nicolson, 1987.
———. "A 'Note' of Interrogation." *Fraser's Magazine* 87, n.s. 7 (May 1873): 567–77.
———. *Notes on Nursing: What It Is and What It Is Not.* London: Harrison, [1859]; New York: D. Appleton, 1860. Reprint New York: Dover, 1969.
———. *Notes on Matters Affecting the Health, Efficiency and Hospital Administration of the British Army.* London: Harrison & Sons, 1858.
———. "A Sub-'Note' of Interrogation." *Fraser's Magazine* 88, n.s. 8 (July 1873): 25–36.
Nutall, Peggy. "The Passionate Statistician." *International Nursing Review* 31, 1 (1984): 24–25.
O'Malley, I. B. *Florence Nightingale: A Study of Her Life Down to the End of the Crimean War.* London: Thornton Butterworth, 1931.
Quinn, E. Vincent and John Prest, eds. *Dear Miss Nightingale: A Selection of Benjamin Jowett's Letters to Florence Nightingale, 1860–1893.* Oxford: Clarendon Press, 1987.
Showalter, Elaine. "Florence Nightingale's Feminist Complaint: Women, Religion, and *Suggestions for Thought.*" *Journal of Women in Culture and Society* 6, 31 (1981): 395–412.
Smith, F. B. *Florence Nightingale: Reputation and Power.* New York: St. Martin's Press, 1982.
Strachey, Lytton. *Eminent Victorians: Cardinal Manning, Florence Nightingale, Dr. Arnold, General Gordon.* London: Chatto and Windus, 1918.
Tooley, Sarah A. *The Life of Florence Nightingale.* London: Cassell, 1910.
Veith, Shirley. "The Recluse: A Retrospective Health History of Florence Nightingale." In Bullough et al., eds., *Florence Nightingale and Her Era: A Collection of New Scholarship,* pp. 75–89.
Vicinus, Martha and Bea Nergaard, eds. *Ever Yours, Florence Nightingale: Selected Letters.* Cambridge, MA: Harvard University Press, 1990.
Welch, Marylouise. "Nineteenth-Century Philosophic Influences on Nightingale's Concept of the Person." *Journal of Nursing History* 1, 2 (1986): 3–11.
Widerquist, Joann. "The Spirituality of Florence Nightingale." *Nursing Research* 41, 1 (Jan/Feb 1992): 49–55.
Woodham-Smith, Cecil Blanche. *Florence Nightingale, 1820–1910.* New York: Mc-Graw-Hill, 1951.

OTHER WORKS

Addinall, Peter. *Philosophy and Biblical Interpretation: A Study in Nineteenth-Century Conflict.* Cambridge: Cambridge University Press, 1991.
Allchin, A. M. *The Silent Rebellion: Anglican Religious Communities, 1845–1900.* London: SCM, 1958.
Altholz, Josef L. "The Mind of Victorian Orthodoxy: Anglican Responses to "Essays and Reviews,' 1860–1864." *Church History* 51 (June 1982): 186–97.

Arnold, Thomas. "Letters on the Social Condition of the Operative Classes." In Arnold, *Miscellaneous Works*, pp. 171–248. London: 1874.

Barth, Karl. *The Theology of Schleiermacher: Lectures at Gottingen, Winter Semester of 1923/24.* Edited by Dietrich Ritschl. Grand Rapids, MI: William B. Eerdman, 1982.

Bicknell, E. J. *A Theological Introduction to the Thirty-Nine Articles of the Church of England.* 3rd edition rev. by H. J. Carpenter. London: Longmans, Green, 1955.

Blackham. H. J. *Six Existentialist Thinkers.* London: Routledge and Kegan Paul, 1952.

Bowen, Desmond. *The Idea of the Victorian Church: A Study of the Church of England, 1833–1889.* Montreal: McGill University Press, 1968.

Broderick, John F., ed. *Documents of Vatican Council I: 1869–1870.* Collegeville, MN: Liturgical Press, n.d.

Buckle, Henry Thomas. *The History of Civilisation in England.* 2 vols. London: John W. Parker, 1857–1861.

Bunsen, Christian von. *Christianity and Mankind.* 7 vols. London: Longman et al., 1854.

———. *The Church of the Future.* 1847.

———. *Egypt's Place in Universal History.* 5 vols. London: Longmans, 1848–67.

———. *God in History.* 3 vols. London: Longmans, 1868–70.

———. *Hippolytus and His Age.* 3 vols. London: Longmans et al., 1852.

———. *Signs of the Times.* London: Smith, Elder, 1856.

Bunsen, Frances Baroness. *Christian Carl Josias Freiherr von Bunsen aus seinem Briefen und nach eigener Erinnerung geschildert.* 3 vols. Leipzig: F. U. Brockhaus, 1868–71.

———. *Memoir of Baron Bunsen, drawn chiefly from the family papers by his widow Frances Baroness Bunsen.* 2 vols. Second edition, abridged and corrected. Philadelphia: J. B. Lippincott, 1869.

Burstyn, Joan N. *Victorian Education and the Ideal of Womanhood.* London: Croom Helm, 1980.

Cashdollar, Charles D. *The Transformation of Theology, 1830–1890: Positivism and Protestant Thought in Britain and America.* Princeton, NJ: Princeton University Press, 1989.

Chadwick, Owen. *The Spirit of the Oxford Movement: Tractarian Essays.* Cambridge: Cambridge University Press.

———. *The Victorian Church.* 2 vols. Third edition. London: Adam and Charles Black, 1971.

Chaudhuri, Nirad C. *Scholar Extraordinary: The Life of Professor the Rt. Hon. Friedrich Max Müller, P.C.* London: Chatto and Windus, 1974.

Clements, Keith. *Friedrich Schleiermacher: Pioneer of Modern Theology.* London: Collins, 1987.

Cockshut, Anthony O. J., ed. *Religious Controversy in Mid-Victorian England.* Newton Abbott, Devon: David and Charles, 1970.

Colenso, John William. *Pentateuch and Book of Joshua Critically Examined.* 1862.

Corsi, Pietro. *Science and Religion: Baden Powell and the Anglican Debate, 1800–1860.* Cambridge: Cambridge University Press, 1988.

Crowther, M. A. *Church Embattled: Religious Controversy in Mid-Victorian England.* Newton Abbot, Devon: David and Charles, 1970.

Davies, Horton. *Worship and Theology in England.* Vol. 3, *From Watts and Wesley to Maurice, 1690–1850.* Princeton, NJ: Princeton University Press, 1961.

Deirdre, David. *Intellectual Women and Victorian Patriarchy: Harriet Martineau, Elizabeth Barrett Browning, George Eliot.* Ithaca, NY: Cornell University Press, 1987.

Distad, N. Merrill. *Guessing at Truth: The Life of Julius Charles Hare (1795–1855).* Shepherdstown, WV: Patmos Press, 1979.

Eckhart, Meister. *Meister Eckhart: The Essential Sermons, Commentaries, Treatises, and Defense.* Trans. Edmund Colledge and Bernard McGinn. New York: Paulist Press, 1981.

Edwards, David Lawrence. *Christian England. Vol. 3: From the Eighteenth Century to the First World War.* Grand Rapids, MI: William B. Eerdmans, 1984.

Ellis, Ieuan. *Seven Against Christ: A Study of "Essays and Reviews".* Leiden:Brill, 1980.

Eliot, George. *The Life of George Eliot as Related in Her Letters and Journals.* Arranged and edited by her husband J. W. Cross. New York: Crowell and Co., 1884.

Froude, James Anthony. *Nemesis of Faith.* London: Chapman, 1849. Reprinted London: Libris, 1988.

Goodwin, C. W. "On the Mosaic Cosmogony." In Jowett, ed., *Essays and Reviews.*

Gray, Robert. *Cardinal Manning: A Biography.* New York: St. Martin's Press, 1985.

Hare, Julius Charles. *The Life and Letters of Frances Baroness Bunsen.* New York: George Routledge, 1879.

Harris, Horton. *David Friedrich Strauss and His Theology.* Cambridge: Cambridge University Press, 1983.

Head, Joseph and S. L. Cranston, comps. *Reincarnation: An East-West Anthology.* Wheaton, Il: Theosophical Publishing House, 1968.

Hill, Michael. *The Religious Order: A Study of Virtuoso Religion and Its Legitimation in the Nineteenth-Century Church of England.* London: Heinemann, 1973.

Hume, David. *Enquiries Concerning Human Understanding and Concerning the Principles of Morals.* 1748.

Huxley, Aldous. *The Perennial Philosophy.* New York: Harper and Row, 1945.

Hinchliff, Peter Bingham. *Benjamin Jowett and the Christian Religion.* Oxford: Clarendon Press, 1987.

Inglis, K. S. "Patterns of Religious Worship in 1851." *Journal of Ecclesiastical History* 11, 1 (1960): 74–86.

Jowett, Benjamin, ed. *Essays and Reviews.* London: John W. Parker and Son, 1860. Reprinted Westmead: Gregg International, 1970.

———. *The Epistles of St. Paul to the Thessalonians, Galatians, Romans.* Second edition. London: John Murray, 1859.

———. "On the Interpretation of Scripture." In *Essays and Reviews.*

———. *The School and Children's Bible.* 1873.

Ker, Ian T. *John Henry Newman: A Biography.* Oxford University Press, 1988.

Macaulay, Thomas Babington. *The History of England.* 5 vols. London: Longmans et al., 1849–1861.

Mackay. *Progress of the Intellect*. London: J. Chapman, 1850.

Malmgren, Gail, ed. *Religion in the Lives of English Women: 1760–1930*. Bloomington: Indiana University Press, 1986.

Mansel, Henry Longueville. *The Limits of Religious Thought Examined*. 1858.

Martineau, Harriet. *The Positive Philosophy of August Comte*. New York: W. Gowans, 1868.

———. *England and Her Soldiers*. 1859.

Martineau, James. *The Rationale of Religious Enquiry*. 1836.

———. *Studies of Christianity; or, Timely Thoughts for Religious Thinkers: A Series of Papers*. Boston: American Unitarian Association, 1858.

Maurice, Frederick Denison. *The Kingdom of Christ; or Hints to a Quaker, Respecting the Principles, Constitution, and Ordinances of the Catholic Church*. 2nd ed. London: J.G.F. & J. Rivington, 1842.

———. *Theological Essays*. Reprinted New York: Harper, 1957.

———. *The Word "Eternal," and the Punishment of the Wicked*. Cambridge: Macmillan and Co., 1853.

McHugh, Paul. *Prostitution and Victorian Social Reform*. New York: St. Martin's Press, 1980.

McIntyre, J. L. *Giordano Bruno*. London: Macmillan, 1903.

Mill, John Stuart. *The Subjection of Women*. Second edition. London: Longmans, 1869. Reprint, edited and with an introduction by Sue Mansfield. Arlington Heights, VA: AHM, 1980.

———. *On Liberty*. 1859.

———. *A System of Logic, Ratiocinative and Inductive, being a connected view of the principles of evidence and the methods of scientific investigation*. 1843. Reprinted Toronto: University of Toronto Press, 1974.

Mitchell, Sally et al., eds. *Victorian Britain: An Encyclopedia*. New York: Garland, 1988.

Moore, James R., ed. *Religion in Victorian Britain*. Vol. 3, *Sources*. Manchester: Manchester University Press, 1988.

Mozley, J. B. *Eight Lectures on Miracles*. 1865.

Müller, Friedrich Max. *Chips from a German Workshop*. 3 vols. New York: Scribner, 1869. Vol. 1 reprinted Chico, CA: Scholars Press, 1985.

———. *The Life and Letters of the Right Honourable Friedrich Max Müller*. 2 vols. London: Kegan Paul, Trench and Co., 1887. Reprinted New York: AMS Press, 1976.

Newman, Francis William. *The Soul*. London, 1849.

Newman, John Henry Cardinal. *Apologia Pro Vita Sua: Being a History of His Religious Views*. 1864. Ed. Martin J. Svaglic. Oxford: Clarendon Press, 1967.

———. "Remarks on Certain Passages in the Thirty-Nine Articles." Tracts for the Times, Tract XC, 1841.

———. "The Miracles of Scripture." In *Two Essays on Biblical and Ecclesiastical Miracles*. London: Pickering and Co., 1881.

———. "The Miracles of Early Ecclesiastical History." In *Two Essays on Biblical and Ecclesiastical Miracles*. London: Pickering and Co., 1881.

Newsome, David. "Newman and the Oxford Movement." In *The Victorian Crisis of Faith*, ed. Anthony Symondson. London: SPCK, 1970.

Norman, Edward R. *The English Catholic Church in the Nineteenth Century*. Oxford: Clarendon Press, 1984.

O'Connell, Marvin R. *The Oxford Conspirators: A History of the Oxford Movement, 1833–1845*. London: University Press of America, 1991.

Oersted, Hans Christian. *The Soul in Nature*. London: H. G. Bohn, 1852.

Owen, Ralph A. D. *Christian Bunsen and Liberal English Theology*. Montpellier, VT: Capital City Press, 1924.

Paley, William. *A View of the Evidences of Christianity. The Works of William Paley*, vol. 2. Boston: Joshua Belcher, 1810.

Pattison, Mark. *Essays by the Late Mark Pattison*. Collected and arranged by Henry Nettleship. Oxford: Clarendon Press, 1879. Reprinted New York: Burt Franklin, 1965.

———. *Memoirs*. London: Macmillan, 1885. Reprinted Gregg International, 1969.

———. "Tendencies of Religious Thought in England, 1688–1750." In Jowett, ed., *Essays and Reviews*.

Pickering, George C. *Creative Malady*. New York: Oxford University Press, 1974.

Powell, Baden. *The Order of Nature: considered in reference to the claims of Revelation*. London: Longman, Brown et al., 1859.

———. "On the Study of the Evidences of Christianity." In Jowett, ed., *Essays and Reviews*.

Preyer, Robert. "Bunsen and the Anglo-American Literary Community in Rome." In *Der Gelehrte Diplomat*, edited by Erich Geldbach. Leiden: Brill, 1980.

Pusey, Edward Bouverie. *An Historical Enquiry into the Probable Causes of the Rationalist Character Lately Predominant in the Theology of Germany*. 1827.

———. *Scriptural Views of Holy Baptism*. Tracts for the Times nos. 67–69. 1835.

Quetelet, Adolphe. *Sur l'homme et la développement de ses facultés: physique sociale*. 1835.

Sanders, Charles Richard. *Coleridge and the Broad Church Movement*. New York: Russell and Russell, 1972.

Schleiermacher, Friedrich. *On Religion: Speeches to Its Cultured Despisers*. Translated by John Oman. Reprinted New York: Harper and Row, 1958.

———. *The Christian Faith*. Ed. H. R. Mackintosh and J. S. Stewart. English translation of the second German edition. Philadelphia: Fortress Press, 1928.

Scott, Walter, ed. and trans. *Hermetica: The Ancient Greek and Latin Writings Which Contain Religious or Philosophic Teachings Attributed to Hermes Trismegistus*. Reprinted Oxford: Clarendon Press, 1924.

Simpson, M. C. M. *Letters and Recollections of Julius and Mary Elizabeth Mohl*. London: Kegan Paul, Trench and Co., 1887.

"Smith, William." Entry in *Dictionary of National Biography*, vol. 53, p. 149

Spinoza, Benedict de. *Tractatus Theologico-politicus*, VI. In *The Chief Works of Benedict de Spinoza*, translated from the Latin, with an introduction by R. H. M. Elwes. New York: Dover, 1951.

Stanley, Arthur P. *Life and Correspondence of Dr. Arnold*. 1844.

Strachey, Ray. *The Cause: A Short History of the Women's Movement in Great Britain*. London: G. Bell, 1928.

Strauss, David Friedrich. *Das Leben Jesu*. 1835.

Summers, Anne. "Ministering Angels." *History Today* 39 (Feb 1989): 31–37.

Temple, Frederick. *Relations Between Religion and Science: Eight Lectures Preached Before the University of Oxford in the Year 1884*. London: Macmillan, 1884; reprinted 1972.

———. "The Education of the World." In Jowett, ed., *Essays and Reviews*.

Thirlwall, Connop. *History of Greece*. 8 vols. 1835–44.

Tulloch, John. *Movements of Religious Thought in Britain During the Nineteenth Century*. New York: C. Scribner's Son, 1885. Reprinted New York: Humanities Press, 1971.

Underhill, Evelyn. *Mysticism: A Study in the Nature and Development of Man's Spiritual Consciousness*. 1911. Twelfth edition reprinted New York: Doubleday, 1988.

Walker, Helen. *Studies in the History of the Statistical Method*. Baltimore: Williams and Wilkins, 1929.

Walkowitz, Judith R. *Prostitution and Victorian Society: Women, Class and the State*. Cambridge: Cambridge University Press, 1980.

Wheeler, Michael. *Death and the Future Life in Victorian Literature and Theology*. Cambridge: Cambridge University Press, 1990.

Wigmore-Beddoes, Dennis G. *Yesterday's Radicals: A Study of the Affinity Between Unitarianism and Broads Church Anglicanism in the Nineteenth Century*. Cambridge: James and Clarke, 1971.

Wilbur, Earl Morse. *A History of Unitarianism. Vol. 2: Transylvania, England, and America*. Cambridge, MA: Harvard University Press, 1952.

Willey, Basil. *Darwin and Butler: Two Versions of Evolution*. New York: Harcourt Brace and Co., 1960.

———. *More Nineteenth Century Studies: A Group of Honest Doubters*. New York: Columbia University Press, 1956.

———. *Nineteenth Century Studies: Coleridge to Matthew Arnold*. London: Chatto and Windus, 1956.

Williams, Rowland. *Christianity and Hinduism: A Dialogue of the Knowledge of the Supreme Lord, in Which are Compared the Claims of Christianity and Hinduism*. Cambridge: Deighton, Bell, 1856.

———. "Bunsen's Biblical Researches." In *Essays and Reviews*. London: John W. Parker and Son, 1860. Reprinted Westmead: Gregg International, 1970.

———. *Lampeter Theology Exemplified in Extracts from the Vice-Principal's Lectures, Letters, and Sermons*. London: Bell and Daldy, 1856.

Williamson, Eugene L. *The Liberalism of Thomas Arnold*. University: University of Alabama Press, 1964.

Wilson, H. B. "Séances Historiques de Genève. The National Church." In Jowett, ed., *Essays and Reviews*.

Woolf, Virginia. *A Room of One's Own*. New York: Harcourt and World, 1929.

Index

University of Pennsylvania Press
STUDIES IN HEALTH, ILLNESS, AND CAREGIVING
Joan E. Lynaugh, General Editor

Barbara Bates. *Bargaining for Life: A Social History of Tuberculosis, 1876–1938*. 1992.
Michael D. Calabria and Janet A. Macrae, editors. Suggestions for Thought *by Florence Nightingale: Selections and Commentaries*. 1994.
Janet Golden and Charles Rosenberg. *Pictures of Health: A Photographic History of Health Care in Philadelphia*. 1991.
Anne Hudson Jones. *Images of Nurses: Perspectives from History, Art, and Literature*. 1987.
June S. Lowenberg. *Caring and Responsibility: The Crossroads Between Holistic Practice and Traditional Medicine*. 1989.
Peggy McGarrahan. *Transcending AIDS: Nurses and HIV Patients in New York City*. 1994.
Elizabeth Norman. *Women at War: The Story of Fifty Military Nurses Who Served in Vietnam*. 1990.
Anne Opie. *There's Nobody There: Community Care of Confused Older People*. 1992.
Elizabeth Brown Pryor. *Clara Barton, Professional Angel*. 1987.
Margarete Sandelowski. *With Child in Mind: Studies of the Personal Encounter with Infertility*. 1993.
Zane Robinson Wolf. *Nurses' Work: The Sacred and The Profane*.
Jacqueline Zalumas. *Caring in Crisis: An Oral History of Critical Care Nursing*. 1994.

This book has been set in Linotron Galliard and Optima. Galliard was designed for Mergenthaler in 1978 by Matthew Carter. Galliard retains many of the features of a sixteenth-century typeface cut by Robert Granjon but has some modifications that give it a more contemporary look. Optima was designed in 1958 for the Stempel Typefoundry by Hermann Zapf. Optima is a very readable sans serif due to the thickening of the letter towards the end, a characteristic of many serif typefaces.